The New Doctor, Patient, Illness Model: Restoring the Authority of the GP Consultation

PETER BAILEY

MB BS BSc DCH DRCOG MRCGP

Freelance General Practitioner, Cambridge

Foreword by

JONATHAN SILVERMAN

Associate Clinical Dean and Director of Communication Studies
School of Clinical Medicine, University of Cambridge, UK
President-elect, European Association for Communication in Healthcare

Radcliffe Publishing
London • New York

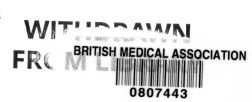

Radcliffe Publishing Ltd
St Mark's House
Shepherdess Walk
London N1 7BQ
United Kingdom

www.radcliffehealth.com

British Library Cataloguing in Publication Data

A catalogue record for this book is available from the British Library.

ISBN-13: 978 184619 898 4

The paper used for the text pages of this book is FSC® certified. FSC (The Forest Stewardship Council®) is an international network to promote responsible management of the world's forests.

Typeset by Darkriver Design, Auckland, New Zealand
Printed and bound by Hobbs the Printers, Totton, Hants, UK

Contents

Foreword

In the last few years, the world of medicine feels to be in constant flux, partly because of rapidly advancing science and technology and partly because of political diktats which have destabilised medicine in the UK through a seemingly constant series of reorganisations. Yet from both the doctor's and the patient's perspective, there is one unchanging beacon in this uncertain world, the consultation. The consultation is everything in medicine, the bedrock on which all else depends. Whatever happens politically, we can be certain that the consultation will remain intact as the vital constant and central element of medical practice. As Sir James Spence said over 60 years ago:

> The real work of a doctor is not an affair of health centres, or laboratories, or hospital beds. Techniques have their place in medicine, but they are not medicine. The essential unit of medical practice is the occasion when, in the intimacy of the consulting room or sick room, a person who is ill, or believes himself to be ill, seeks the advice of a doctor whom he trusts. This is a consultation, and all else in the practice of medicine derives from it.

All of this makes Peter Bailey's heartfelt exposition of his own personal journey through consulting over the last 30 years in general practice incredibly apposite. This book *The New Doctor, Patient, Illness Model: Restoring the Authority of the GP Consultation* is different from many recent texts on consulting or clinical communication. It does not attempt to be a learned research-based treatise. Instead, Peter has written a labour of love, a personal historical account of his own learning from a lifetime of consulting with patients. The manuscript oozes Peter's desire to record what he has struggled with over all these years as a highly skilled practitioner.

As you read it, you are aware of the personal efforts to achieve the very best from each elusive and fleeting consultation. And you are introduced to the many and varied influences that have shaped Peter's thoughts over the years.

Being of the same age as Peter, I resonated with the historical un-rolling of influential ideas from people such as Balint, Bendix, Pendleton and recognised how the thoughts of local doyens of general practice could lastingly form one's opinions and attitudes.

Yet this isn't only history. Peter has spent a considerable time thinking about how to put all these influences together in a model which enhances our understanding of the consultation. He has taken Balint's original concept of doctor, patient and illness and has produced a diagrammatic representation where the overlaps become all-important. These overlaps allow the reader to understand the importance of the relationship between doctor and patient and the different story of the illness brought to the consultation by the doctor and the patient. His diagram establishes the influence of the social context of the doctor, the patient and the illness.

And at the heart of the diagram lies the central overlap which Peter calls the authority of the consultation. I have debated with Peter whether authority is the right choice of word. Even though I understood what Peter was meaning, *'the authority that is generated by the patient and the doctor working together; through shared understanding and mutual respect'*, I was concerned that the reader would hear the word 'authority' and think of it in terms of a paternalistic approach to medicine, the exact opposite of what Peter is espousing. To me, centrality would be more appropriate. But Peter is sure that it is indeed the *authority of the consultation* that needs to be re-established in this particularly difficult era in medicine, and that it is through listening, understanding, respect, partnership and shared understanding that the doctor and the patient can together move forward, with the *'patient as author of their own life'*.

Peter's conclusions from a lifetime of working dramatically mirror the research evidence that has accumulated over the last 30 years concerning doctor–patient communication. The approaches that he advocates are completely in accord with modern developments in patient-centred/relationship-centred medicine and the evolving field of shared decision-making.

There have been many recent developments in the structure of general practice which have placed intense pressure on the consultation. While the patient's agenda should be foremost, high-quality prevention, chronic disease management, and health behaviour modification have all become important considerations. The computer has established itself as an essential third participant in the consultation. These influences have all had a tendency to push GPs towards a directing rather than a guiding style. Peter's thoughtful model will hopefully enable future practitioners of medicine to argue against any retrograde move towards paternalism and authoritarianism. His book carefully explains why the consultation needs to be re-established as the central endeavour of us all, the means towards achieving shared understanding, placing patients in charge of their own destiny and enabling doctors to have fulfilling and lasting careers.

Jonathan Silverman
Associate Clinical Dean and Director of Communication Studies
School of Clinical Medicine, University of Cambridge, UK
President-elect, European Association for
Communication in Healthcare
January 2014

Preface

This book is about authority. Not the authoritarianism of the arrogant doctor or the consumerism of the 'I know my rights' patient, but the authority that is generated by the patient and the doctor working together; through shared understanding and mutual respect. It is about the authority of the consultation – a consultation that takes account of all the necessary facts and perspectives. The outcome of a consultation with this authority is a way forward for the patient that meets their needs. The general overview or 'Synoptic View' that I am presenting is a new way of looking at the familiar triad of Doctor, Patient and Illness. It provides a template onto which the information elicited during the consultation can be collected for synthesis allowing better management plans to be framed. Such plans are owned and understood by the patient and the doctor. Chosen together, adherence to the plan is more likely and outcomes and satisfaction improve.

I have had help and encouragement from many people. Jonathan Silverman's advice saved me from some important errors and omissions – any remaining are all my own. My constant friends Peter Kaye, Josephine Fagan and Tobi Megchild have shown great faith when my own has flagged, and my colleagues and patients at Monkfield Medical Practice in Cambourne have borne with fortitude my experimentation with these ideas.

Peter Bailey
Cambridge
January 2014

About the Author

Dr Peter Bailey is a Cambridge-based, freelance general practitioner. He was a principal in general practice from 1984 until 2012. He has experience of teaching medical students and has been a general practitioner trainer. He now undertakes freelance sessional work and runs a vasectomy service. He is an appraiser and is also a coach and mentor for general practitioners.

> *When people see this book, they will think that you are some sort of expert communicator.*
>   *Well, you're ****ing not!*

> Author's wife, personal communication, 2013

Acknowledgements

Reference 3 reproduced by kind permission of the Royal College of General Practitioners. Working Party of the Royal College of General Practitioners. *The Future General Practitioner*. London: Royal College of General Practitioners; 1972.

Reference 8 reproduced with permission of John Wiley & Sons, Inc. Stacey R. *Managing the Unknowable: strategic boundaries between order and chaos in organizations*. San Francisco, CA: Jossey-Bass; 1992.

Reference 11 used by permission of Alfred A. Knopf, an imprint of the Knopf Doubleday Publishing Group, a division of Random House LLC. Excerpt from *Chance and Necessity* by Jaques Monod and translated by Austryn Wainhouse, translation © 1971 by Alfred A. Knopf, a division of Random House LLC. All rights reserved. Any third party use of this material, outside of this publication, is prohibited. Interested parties must apply directly to Random House LLC for permission.

Reference 13 reprinted with the permission of Simon and Schuster Publishing Group from *The Road Less Traveled* by M. Scott Peck M.D, © 1978 M. Scott Peck.

Reference 78 reproduced with the permission of Elsevier from Michael Balint, *The Doctor, His Patient and the Illness* (2nd ed., London: Churchill Livingstone; 2000), p. 1.

Reference 87 reproduced by permission from Enid Balint and JS Norell, editors, *Six Minutes for the Patient: interactions in general practice consultation* (London: Tavistock Publications; 1973), p. 151.

Reference 88 reproduced by permission from Enid Balint and JS Norell, editors,

Six Minutes for the Patient: interactions in general practice consultation (London: Tavistock Publications; 1973), p. 21.

Reference 94 reprinted by permission of Houghton Mifflin Harcourt Publishing Company. All rights reserved. Excerpt from 'The Dry Salvages' from *Four Quartets* by TS Eliot. © 1941 by TS Eliot. © renewed 1969 by Esme Valerie Eliot.

Reference 116 reproduced with permission from Naidoo P, Monkley C. *Consultations Skills for the New MRCGP: practice cases for the CSA and COT*. Banbury. © 2012 Scion Publishing Ltd.

Part One

The Synoptic View of the Consultation

INTRODUCTION

It is a precious jewel to be plain
Sometimes in shell the Orient's pearls we find:-
Of others take a sheaf, of me a grain, of me a grain.

John Dowland, 'Fine Knacks for Ladies'
Lute song from the *Second Book of Airs*[1]

Synoptic: *Pertaining to or forming a synopsis; furnishing a general view of some subject*

Oxford English Dictionary[2]

The consultation model presented in this book could be likened to the picture on the box of a difficult jigsaw puzzle. The consultation is endlessly complex and humans are very difficult to understand. Each of us lives our life in the centre of our own private universe of thought and feeling. Reaching out from that privacy and connecting with others is what gives our lives meaning. Our lives are enriched when we communicate and impoverished when we are unable to do so.

1

SCIENCE, ART AND TRUTH

> In General Practice, all the information about the patient and the illness which the doctor is prepared to recognise has to be accepted as a communication with many meanings. On the other hand, the interpretation of this information, the process of testing hypotheses and solving problems, demands the intellectual discipline of the scientific method. Much therefore will be demanded of the future GP. He will need to acquire the approach to man which stems from science – both biological and behavioural – as well as the flair, imagination and compassion, the sense of tragedy and comedy, which characterize the arts.
>
> Working Party of the Royal College of General Practitioners[3]

THE DOCTOR AS HEALER

> It is curious that our power, and what we do as individual doctors to make people better – which is what many people value most in us – seem to get left out of our study of the consultation . . . At times of illness, crisis, loss or threat we all need attention, sympathy and support – indeed, a bit of loving approval. To be assured we have value and worth, that things may not be quite so awful as they feel, that there are features that are positive in what seems like an overwhelmingly negative situation, to have our intrinsic qualities objectively affirmed – these are universal human needs which fall to us as doctors to fulfil. Whether we like it or not, and find it embarrassing to talk about it ourselves, a primary task for us as doctors is to provide this: we are the healers, and society, and its individual members, need us.
>
> Richard Westcott[4]

The hospital model was the foundation of my medical training, but I had already been inspired by the example of my own family's general practitioner. I had seen at first hand the way in which he managed my mother's anxiety when she called him to see my feverish sister. I knew that how you talk to patients is at least as important as what you say to them. I knew that there was much more to learn about communication than what I was seeing on consultant ward rounds. As a medical student I decided to look for a different approach and was fortunate to meet Dr Max Meyer, a GP who worked in Islington. His surgeries were filled with people who did not seem to have any disease or illness that I could recognise. They came to share their lives with him, the heartache of the human predicament of birth, love, loss, betrayal, courage and suffering – everything. He listened to them and thought about them. He would tell me stories about them after they had left and it was clear to me that they felt less alone having been met and understood a little. Of course, he would treat hypertension and diabetes and chest infections as well, but here was healing, in action.

CHAPTER 1

The Puzzle and the Picture: Introducing the Synoptic View

The fool doth think he is wise, but the wise man knows himself to be a fool.

William Shakespeare, *As You Like It* (act 5, scene 1)[5]

Since I qualified in 1979, I have participated in more than 200 000 consultations. I would like to offer a fresh perspective of what happens in a consultation – a general overview or 'synoptic' view. Consultation is not a linear process. It does not have a clear beginning, middle and end. Many of the elements are present even before the patient enters the room. The consultation is better thought of as recursive, or perhaps as a spiral, working towards meeting a patient's needs.

Here, then, is a new way of looking at the consultation. I have devised a simple and easily remembered diagram (as outlined in Figures 1–3 in this chapter) that illuminates the richly complex process.

My starting point was the title of Michael Balint's book *The Doctor, His Patient and the Illness*[6] – a title taken from Hippocrates.[7] This title outlines the three main protagonists in the consultation, although each plays a different role in the consulting room – each has an independent existence, separate from the other contributors. The narrative that emerges as the three interact is the stuff of the consultation. The deepest purpose of the consultation is meeting the patient's needs, and I would argue that that is nearly always achieved by seeking to enhance the patient's autonomy. With this as my guiding principle, I looked at the consultation from a storytelling perspective to see how the process can be facilitated and understood.

Box 1

The key to success lies in the creative activity of making new maps, not in the imitative following and refining of existing ones.

Ralph Stacey, *Managing the Unknowable*[8]

In the quotation shown in Box 1, Ralph Stacey[9] makes it clear that the story of the consultation cannot be written in advance. That it why the Synoptic View of the consultation can help to orientate us in the dizzying turns and the blind alleys of the consultation. It is a guide to the nature of the unfolding narratives rather than any sort of prediction of what will be in them. Therefore, it is not prescriptive of tasks for the doctor, since these must necessarily emerge from the stories.

Drawing the protagonists as overlapping circles produces a diagram as shown in Figure 1.

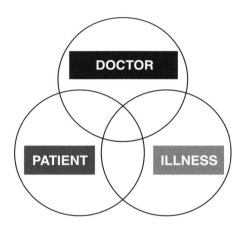

FIGURE 1 The doctor, the patient and the illness

The overlaps between the three domains represent three quite distinct narratives. Each represents a story waiting to unfold. Each story needs time and attention spent on it if the goal of the consultation is to be achieved.

The three domains are:
1. the patient's story of the illness (which often focuses on subjective symptoms, thoughts and observations)
2. the doctor's story of the illness illness (which often focuses on diseases and organs, pathology and function)

3. the doctor–patient relationship.

The central overlap where all three circles intersect represents the holy grail of consulting. Herein lies the right diagnosis, the best treatment, the patient with improved autonomy, shared understanding and all the other outcomes sought by GP gurus over the years. We are familiar with the idea of patient-centred medicine and doctor-centred medicine. What I am arguing for is *consultation-centred* medicine. A good consultation leads to outcomes that match need. These outcomes are authoritative because they respect the realities of the three protagonists. I am proposing a model that establishes the *authority of the consultation*.

The diagram now looks like that shown in Figure 2.

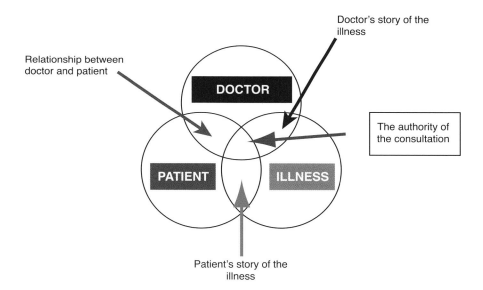

FIGURE 2 The stories within the consultation

The consultation does not occur in isolation, in a social vacuum. Both the doctor and the patient know their social roles. Their interactions are patterned and constrained by expectation, habit and fashion. Additionally, disease and illness themselves are not free of social meaning and significance.

There is a social boundary around the consultation and this can be represented by a triangle around the protagonists. Each aspect – illness, doctor and patient – has a unique social context, but all share in society. The conclusion reached in the shared understanding at the close of the consultation will reflect the mores and customs of that context. Now the diagram looks like that shown in Figure 3.

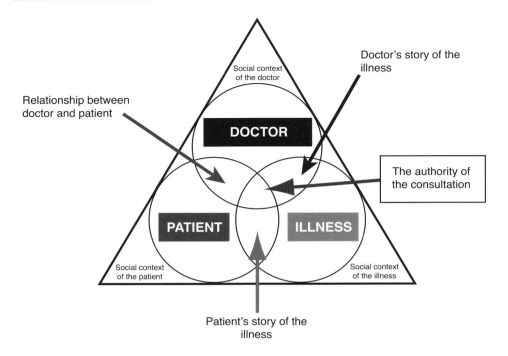

FIGURE 3 The Synoptic View of the consultation

This is the 'picture on the jigsaw puzzle box' that I have called the Synoptic View of the consultation.

Every consultation is a unique opportunity for meeting a person in his or her predicament, for making a difference. No map or diagram can encompass the complexity of the journey that results, but perhaps the model presented can steady the nerves and help to orientate the physician as the process unfolds. Just like the picture on the box of a fiendishly difficult jigsaw puzzle, this model can help you to see where the pieces fit. We find it almost impossible to perceive what we are *not* looking for, to observe what we do *not* expect to find. The consultation model can help you to perceive more in your consultations, to allocate what you notice correctly and to get closer to the right diagnosis and management. Using this model can enhance the authority of your consultations.

CHAPTER 2

The Doctor

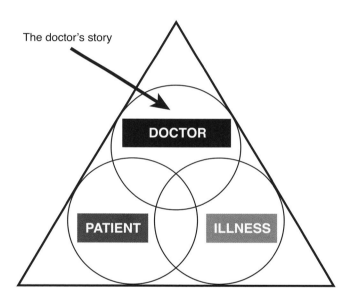

The doctor's story

FIGURE 4 The doctor

My thoughts about why I am a doctor have matured over the years, but my early experiences set my path and prompted me into general practice – the coalface of medicine. It is in general practice that unnamed illness and complexity seek to be understood. In 1972 a Royal College of General Practitioners document asked:

> A woman of 30 presents to her GP with her three year old daughter. The child is irritable and badly behaved. She is crying constantly during the night and keeping the parents awake. Her elderly mother is due to visit, and she is worried what her mother will think to find the house and child in such a state. But her

main worry is that her husband is waking in the night with abdominal pains – could it be an ulcer?[10]

Box 2

When I was 10 years old, the second eldest of six children, there was little that could disturb the equanimity of my mother. She had dealt with all our childhood illnesses, cooked and cleaned and catered through the impecunious fifties, taught us our tables and our table manners and encouraged our curiosity.

Then Angela, one of my sisters, became unwell. 'Could it be scarlet fever or even meningitis?' my mother wondered. This was my first experience of seeing my mother distracted and anxious, even frightened. Our GP was called.

He arrived at the house, and examined my sister on the sofa in our sitting room. Gathered outside the door, we children strained to hear what was said. At last the doctor got up to leave and we scampered to the stairs as my mother thanked him and said goodbye. It was just tonsillitis. My mother's relief suffused her face and she smiled to us. Her frown was gone and she was brisk and efficient and comforting, back in charge.

How had this visitor achieved this miracle? What skill and craft did he employ to leave this gift of relief of fear with my mother? I wanted to know. I wanted to become a doctor.

I told my grandmother I wanted to become a doctor. She gave me a kiss and half a crown. Now I was sure!

This is the very stuff of life. As a GP I have the privilege of being invited inside such stories with the hope that together we may be able to make the predicament more manageable, reduce suffering and anxiety and improve autonomy.

There is a common triad of characteristics or personality traits in members of the helping professions, especially prevalent in healthcare workers who frequently exhibit:

- high levels of perfectionism
- an exaggerated sense of responsibility
- guilt.

Each of these traits has a useful side to it. You would wish your oncologist to calculate your chemotherapy dose correctly – perfectionism would seem a desirable characteristic under such circumstances. Or during a change in shift in the accident and emergency department you would want your major trauma dealt with effectively and you would be glad if the cardiothoracic surgeon who began the repair of your great vessels stayed on until the job was finished. Or perhaps after a failure in the care of your grandmother you would want the ward manager where she died to conduct a thorough review of what went wrong, motivated by guilt for the mishandling of her care.

However, all too frequently such traits lead to trouble. Perfectionism leads to disillusionment; exaggerated responsibility leads to exhaustion, and marital breakdown and neglect of children; guilt leads to demoralisation, drugs, alcohol and suicide.

So where is balance to be found? As far as the general practice consultation is concerned, I suggest that it lies with the authority found in the centre of the Synoptic View. When proper recognition of the stories of the doctor, the patient and the illness is achieved, the shared understanding that emerges frees the patient from unnecessary anxiety, liberates the doctor from authoritarianism and inappropriate responsibility and unites them both in the struggle to make sense of symptoms, disease and illness. It helps them to face the ultimate inevitability of death and decay just a little less alone than they would otherwise have been.

This common understanding of the human condition can be put to good use in the consultation. It can be the source of exceptionally helpful intuition. You can use your instinctive, uncensored first impressions to inform your understanding of your patient and your interactions with them. As your patient comes through your door, make a mental note of three 'first impression' adjectives. Use your (non-politically correct) antennae to sense something about your patient and allow a prejudiced opinion to surface briefly in your mind.

Here are some recent ones of mine:
- striking, confident and commanding
- thin, tense and preoccupied
- despondent, grey and anxious
- challenging, angry and impatient
- overweight, timid and browbeaten
- exhausted, wary and sad.

There is a very strong probability that you will not be alone in your initial reaction to your patient. There is a real chance that your intuition and first impressions can tell you something about the way your patient habitually experiences the world. He will be projecting something of his belief about himself. You receive it using your antennae, sensing something of his life and interactions. You can hold on to these impressions as extra information as he unfolds the narrative of his illness to you, enabling you to make a richer judgement about the diagnosis.

An important benefit of this technique is that it can make manifest some of your prejudices that might otherwise remain buried in the unconscious, where they remain capable of sabotaging the consultation, leading you to treat your patient in a stereotyped way. A prejudice unrecognised has much more power than one that is acknowledged. If you allow the distortion of any judgemental feelings about your patients to surface, you can deal with them and channel your insight for the patient's benefit. Unacknowledged prejudice subverts your behaviour. You may even damage your patient as you overstep ethical boundaries.

CHAPTER 3

The Patient

The ancient covenant is in pieces; man knows at last that he is alone in the universe's unfeeling immensity, out of which he emerged only by chance. His destiny is nowhere spelled out, nor is his duty. The kingdom above or the darkness below; it is for him to choose.

J Monod, *Chance and Necessity*[11]

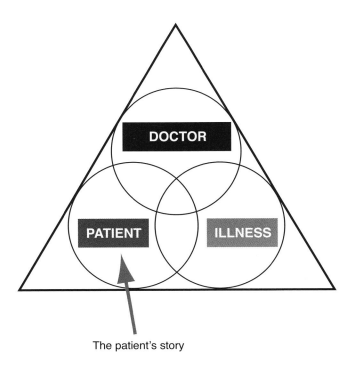

The patient's story

FIGURE 5 The patient

What is it to be a patient? The word implies passivity, suffering and waiting. The patient has sought help because his or her resources no longer meet their need. They have made an assessment of their predicament, their symptoms of disease and decided to look to you, the doctor.

They will have telephoned the practice and negotiated with the receptionist, who has the unenviable task of rationing the doctor's appointments. In a 'free at the point of use' system, demand management is achieved through waiting. In a fee-paying system, demand management is achieved through cost and competition to supply. They will have had to spend resource, either of time or money, in order to have reached you and will want to get value from the consultation.

They will have sat in your waiting room. Waiting is an opportunity for preparation, reflection and imagination. Symptoms, disease and illness are often accompanied by anxiety. Gathered together with other patients, they will have pondered, perhaps chatted with acquaintances, and worried.

Perhaps their underlying question is: 'What does it all mean?' They may be struggling to make sense of illness and birth and death and relationships. They will (whether explicitly or not) have a philosophy, a world view that they have constructed to make an arbitrary and contingent world seem less random.

Box 3

Try to Discover your Patient's Philosophy
Everyone has an explicit or implicit set of ideas and beliefs about the essential nature of the world. This can be considered as the person's philosophy. The patient consciously or unconsciously brings this set of beliefs and ideas to the consultation.

As a schoolboy I happened across a copy of Jacques Monod's book *Chance and Necessity*[12] In it he asserts that everything that happens must be 'either the result of all the antecedent events, however minute and therefore *inevitable and necessary*, or must be the result of the merest *chance* when all other factors are equally balanced.' For a Roman Catholic boy like me, brought up on free will, sin and inescapable death, judgement, heaven and hell, this was a major disturbance to my world view (and one from which I have never fully recovered).

You too may have been brought up with a particular view of causation, or perhaps you have never really thought about it much. Your patients will be in the same position. It is important to discover what their underlying assumptions are. It would be helpful to make your own beliefs explicit for yourself too.

M Scott Peck, in his book *The Road Less Travelled*,[13] makes this point:

> find out your patients' religions even if they say they don't have any.

. . . the fact of the matter is that everyone has an explicit or an implicit set of ideas and beliefs as to the essential nature of the world. Do patients envision the universe as basically chaotic and without meaning so that it is only sensible for them to grab whatever little pleasure they can whenever it is available? Do they see the world as a dog-eat-dog place where ruthlessness is essential for survival? Or do they see it as a nurturing sort of place in which something good will always turn up and in which they need not fret much about the future? Or a place that owes them a living no matter how they conduct their lives? Or a universe of rigid law in which they will be struck down and cast away if they step even slightly out of line?

Illness, disease and distress do not happen in a vacuum. We all try to make sense of what happens to us. Getting an understanding of your patient's philosophy (or 'religion' as Peck calls it) will allow you to make a better connection with him or her. The word 'religion' derives from the Latin *religare*, meaning 'to reconnect with'.

Reaching agreement and the right diagnosis must accommodate the patient's perceptions of causation. If you miss this step, adherence to any plan will be compromised.

Box 4

Our View of the World

In the American Museum of Natural History in New York there is a display that aims to help visitors to understand their place in the universe. Suspended in the centre of an enormous room there is an 87-foot aluminium sphere.

The sphere holds the Hayden Planetarium. It is big enough to hold an audience of hundreds. Around the room at the level of the equator of the sphere there is a walkway. Every few yards there is a display board that uses the size of the sphere to help understand the scale of another object. For example, one board says: 'If the Hayden Sphere were a red blood cell, then this 4-inch model would be the size of a rhinovirus'; at the next display one would see: 'If the Hayden Sphere were a rhinovirus, then this 2-inch model would be the size of a hydrogen atom'. At the start of the display we see the size of the Sphere compared with the size of the known universe, with our home cluster of galaxies an insignificant dot.

The display overwhelms the mind and prompts the observer to ponder his or her own insignificance as stardust whirling through space and time.

CHAPTER 4

The Illness

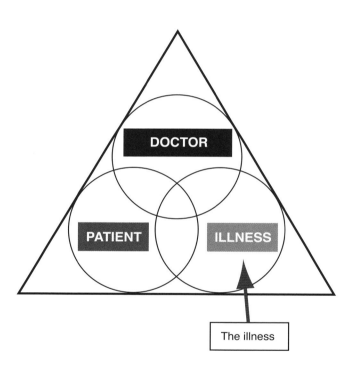

FIGURE 6 The illness

The World Health Organization declares in its constitution that health is a state of complete physical, mental and social well-being and not merely the absence of disease or infirmity.[14]

Are we ill if we are not healthy?

Box 5

The Constitution of the World Health Organization[15]
The following principles are basic to the happiness, harmonious relations and security of all peoples:
- Health is a state of complete physical, mental and social well-being and not merely the absence of disease or infirmity.
- The enjoyment of the highest attainable standard of health is one of the fundamental rights of every human being without distinction of race, religion, political belief, economic or social condition.

In the 1980s a new perspective emerged which looked at the difference between disease and illness. Ian McWhinney, an English physician who later became Professor of Family Medicine in Canada at the University of Western Ontario, described the importance of understanding the enormous difference between the physician's perspective of disease as dysfunction in the organs of the body and the patient's perspective of illness as symptoms indicating dysfunction in health and wellbeing.[16]

At any given moment a significant proportion of the population will have symptoms and a small proportion will seek the advice of a health professional. Some of these seekers will have diseases and a lucky few will receive healthcare that meets their needs.

Illness is a social construct, a meaning placed upon the experience of symptoms by individuals in their social settings.

Diseases are real.

They exist independently of human attempts at understanding and classification. It is only now (in evolutionary terms) that an organism, *Homo sapiens*, has evolved the capacity to speculate on its finitude and ultimate destination and stand apart and contemplate demise and death. We struggle to give meaning to disease and to contain it through naming it and classifying it. Illness is an experience but disease is a phenomenon (a feature of matter, energy or space-time) that is present whether we are there to perceive it or not.

We have all had the jolting experience of realising that the person in front of us is doomed as the diagnosis emerges from the consultation. All physicians know that in the end death wins.

Our atoms are stardust and our universe tends towards chaos. The miracle of our local part of the universe is that complexity has emerged and become sentient for a time. However, we are relentlessly pulled back towards stardust, a fact recognised in the burial service: 'Ashes to ashes, dust to dust'.[17]

That inevitable process involves disease. There is apoptosis and senescence, damage and cancer and decay, and, above all, attack from other organisms intent on their own survival, trying to get a leg up from the energy stored inside us to promote their own success.

Whatever our world view, our level of insight and intelligence, philosophy or culture, we will end. The inevitable decline towards death is characterised by disease. Disease then is its own story. It existed before us and it is likely that it will persist after us. Medicine is the story of the struggle with disease and death, seeking to mitigate the suffering and maintain autonomy.

Box 6

Avoid Imposing Your Own World View
Patient: Pardon, doctor?
Doctor: I said you're WASTING AWAY, Mrs Gilbert, you're turning back to DUST . . .

There is a concept in game theory that is of relevance here and is known as the **locus of control** – used to understand the factors that determine the outcome of activities such as chess or tennis. Skill is internal to the player, while chance and the opponent's skill are external. The probability of success is related to the degree of skill, and the locus of control is said to be internal if the level of skill is high and external if outside factors predominate.

It has been observed that the outcome of a challenge to health is commonly attributed to internal factors such as the choice of a healthy lifestyle, or to external factors such as the quality of the doctor, or to chance. Some patients tend to see themselves as passive, with the locus of health control lying outside themselves; others believe they have the responsibility to deal with their illnesses and have the locus of health control within themselves.

The Synoptic View of the consultation helps the doctor and the patient to understand where the locus of control lies at any given moment and to make an informed choice about where it belongs. Additional resources may be required to enable the patient to shift the locus towards him- or herself – to become more autonomous.

Box 7

Health Locus of Control

Consider a patient with diabetes lapsing into a coma from hypoglycaemia. Once the patient is unconscious, the locus of control is clearly not within the patient's will but lies with the illness. If help does not arrive, the patient risks injury or even death. When the doctor arrives the locus of control moves to the doctor but remains external to the patient. After administration of carbohydrates and glucagon the patient recovers and then has the opportunity to take responsibility for managing his or her diabetes differently in order to prevent a recurrence. The health locus of control can move back to the patient. If this is to be successful it requires the patient to understand the causes of hypoglycaemia and the strategies for reducing the risk of recurrence. Given time and encouragement, information and resources, the health locus of control becomes internal and the patient experiences an increase in his or her autonomy. Insufficient time and resource will leave the patient dependent on the doctor, recurrences are more likely and the disease will intrude upon the patient's life with a consequent reduction in autonomy.

CHAPTER 5

The Patient's Story of the Illness: Fractals

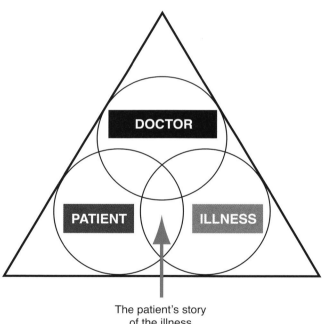

The patient's story
of the illness

FIGURE 7 The patient's story of the illness

To see a world in a Grain of Sand
And Heaven in a wild flower
Hold Infinity in the palm of your hand
And Eternity in an hour.

William Blake, 'Auguries of Innocence' (1803)[18]

How detailed is the patient's story likely to be? This is rather like asking: 'How long is the coastline of Britain?' It depends how you look. A geographic out-line looks similar at nearly all magnifications, so you cannot guess its scale by its contour. If you take all the ins and outs of every rock and sand grain, the answer to the coastline question is: 'It's almost infinite!' Similarly, with a patient's history there is really no limit to how much detail you might seek in the story he or she is telling. You will find that every little detail can be opened up into more cycles of storytelling with ever more richness of history and lay-ers of meaning and echo.

This idea derives from the work of Benoît Mandelbrot, a Polish-born French mathematician working in America for IBM, who in 1967 published a paper in *Science* called 'How Long is the Coast of Britain? Statistical Self-Similarity and Fractional Dimension.'[19] The concept came to be known by the term 'fractal' (from the Latin meaning broken). Fractals are phenomena that are self-similar at various scales of magnification with simple and recursive definitions. You may not know what a fractal is, but you will definitely recognise one when you see one. Many real-life objects or phenomena such as clouds, coastlines, trees and stock market fluctuations have fractal-like properties. Patterns are repeated as you examine fractals in more detail and the particular rules that govern the fractal give it a recognisable and reliable form. The branching of a willow tree, for instance, follows fractal rules and thus, while every willow tree is different, all willow trees are self-similar. Mandelbrot wrote and lectured engagingly about his ideas and they have entered popular culture and contributed to the emergence of chaos theory. Mathematical figures of great beauty and complex-ity that are capable of infinite magnification result from fractal mathematics.

The pictures that follow are of a mathematical pattern known as the Mandelbrot set. This is an iterative function in which the answer to a sum is fed back into the equation so that a new result is produced. Very simple start-ing conditions can lead to startling complexity and very beautiful patterns. The pattern is capable of infinite magnification and it is self-similar, although never identical at all magnifications.

This property is similar to the patient's story. Infinite detail lies beneath the surface of the consultation and histories often contain recurring patterns or themes. It is all too easy to get distracted by a bit of the pattern that interests the doctor and miss something of importance elsewhere. You need help in deciding where to look and it is important to have an overview of the whole before deciding what the diagnosis is. However, you will take forever if you are not selective. The patient will guide you to the right areas.

Like snowflakes (another example of fractal patterns), consultations are self-similar but infinitely varied. Diversity is the joy and beauty of the consulta-tion, and seen in this light nothing is trivial or boring! The bread and butter of

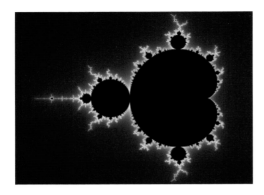

An overview of the Mandelbrot set is equivalent to the rehearsed story of the patient as he presents: 'I am feeling depressed again'.

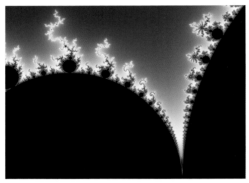

Further exploration of the history reveals that the patient is 'run down' and 'vulnerable to every infection going'. This is the equivalent of magnifying the Mandelbrot image.

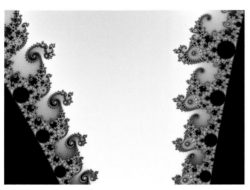

Further magnification reveals that the patient is bullied at work.

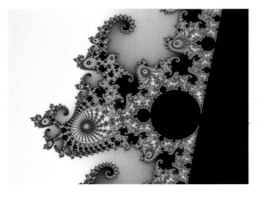

More magnification still and the patient says that he lacks assertiveness . . .

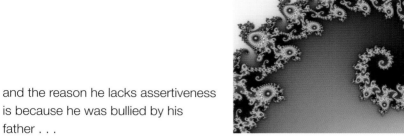

and the reason he lacks assertiveness is because he was bullied by his father . . .

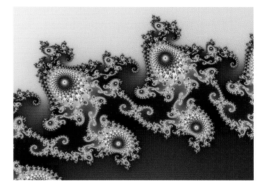

and his father was himself abused while he was in care in a children's home . . .

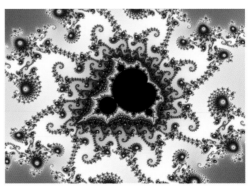

where he was placed because his unmarried mother was unable to look after him . . .

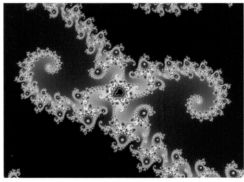

because she suffered from depression because . . . (and so on).

general practice – sore throats and back pain, anxiety and depression, disease and the fear of disease, antenatal and palliative care – all become a privileged exploration of the exquisite patterns of human life.

There is an endless amount of detail that can be elicited from a patient by facilitating more and more storytelling. Stories have different meanings at different levels. Different stories will have differing levels of complexity hidden within them.

The task for the doctor is to guide the patient into the right amount of storytelling. Too much and the doctor is swamped by a mass of detail that cannot be assimilated or understood; too little and the problem is not recognisable. Your patient will help you in deciding how much storytelling is useful, but you will have to use your professional training to steer gently from time to time.

CHAPTER 6

The Patient's Story of the Illness: Narrative

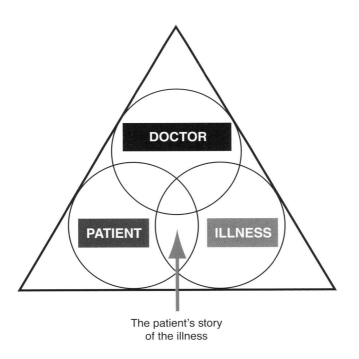

The patient's story
of the illness

FIGURE 8 The patient's story of the illness

'But wait a bit,' the Oysters cried
'Before we have our chat;
For some of us are out of breath,
And all of us are fat!'
'No hurry!' said the Carpenter.
They thanked him much for that.

Lewis Carroll, *Tweedledum and Tweedledee*[20]

When the patient enters your consulting room and starts to speak he or she will probably launch into a rehearsed speech. They may have been practising while they have been waiting to see you. They have probably rehearsed it a few times with the other people with whom they may have discussed their problem.

The language that the patient uses may be somewhat stilted because they will have tried to put the problem in a form that they think will 'please' you. Their presentation may convey little of their own beliefs and ideas because they know that they have come to you (the 'great shaman') for assistance.

The patient's speech will help to define the general territory of the consultation and you will soon begin to feel yourself settling comfortably into professional problem-solving mode.

AT THIS STAGE, RESIST SPEAKING AT ALL COSTS! GIVE YOUR PATIENT 'WAIT TIME'

The concept of wait time is well established in educational theory. Mary Rowe has written and researched extensively in this field. The research establishes the usefulness of pausing after asking questions, giving people time to think, rather than rushing in with a suggestion, an answer or another question.[21]

Whatever your discipline in medicine you will have been trained to ask questions – to take a history. The purpose of the history (you have been told) is to allow you to fit the patient's story into your classification of disorders so that you can bring your enormous diagnostic skill and treatment prowess into play and effect a wondrous cure.

All your training will now have been activated. You will be testing algorithms in your mind, recognising patterns, remembering protocols and allocating patients to clinical trials in your head.

REMEMBER: *DO NOTHING*

Something significant is about to happen.

This is no time for history taking. This is a time for storytelling!

Allow the patient to tell their story. Encourage the story to go the way it needs to, through prompts and encouragement, but as far as possible without questions.

> *Break, break, break*
> *On thy cold gray stones, O Sea!*
> *And I would that my tongue could utter*
> *The thoughts that arise in me.*
>
> Alfred Tennyson, 1st Baron Tennyson (1842)[22]

You now have a rare opportunity. You can do something that allows you to convert the patient in front of you from mere patient into an individual, a fully rounded human being, who, like you, is trying to make sense of what is happening to them.

Hidden just below the story the patient has told you (the rehearsed story) lies the whole richness of their human experience and the unedited version of their story. All that has gone into him or her, nature and nurture, has culminated in this moment of consultation. If you hold your nerve and prompt gently, you can have the privilege of dipping into your patient's experience.

Most people are bursting to tell their story. Finding a competent listener is like finding a precious jewel.

All you need to do to start the next phase of the consultation is to nudge the patient. You have already proved that you are a good listener. Your patient is predisposed to trust you because of your role, and now you have demonstrated that you are paying attention too.

So, how do you nudge your patient into telling you their unrehearsed story?

Simple: just ask a question in a way that cannot be answered with a simple yes or no. Everyone has his or her favourites. You might try one like:

> I see. Tell me a little more about it all . . .

or (my preferred option):

> Hmm. Take me right back to the very beginning and tell me what happened . . .

Unfailingly, your patient will now launch into the everyday speech version of their story. There will be much more detail in the story and the language will their own. There will be much less editing and other people are likely to figure more. Feelings and ideas may be beginning to creep in.

At this stage of the consultation you don't have to be clever or think very hard. You just have to listen.

Box 8

This is not a time for impressing your patient with how clever you are. It is a time for finding out how clever your patient is.

Listen actively during the retelling of the story.

IDEAS, CONCERNS AND EXPECTATIONS

In 1984, David Pendleton and colleagues in Oxford introduced the notion of looking specifically for the patient's ideas, concerns and expectations. While waiting for the doctor, you can be sure that your patient has been speculating about their illness.[23] They will have formed an opinion regarding the nature of the problem and its possible causes. They will have considered a range of possibilities, some of which may be trivial but some that may be potentially fatal. From these ideas and concerns there flows a many-branched tree of possibilities, and they will have expectations for what you might say and do in the course of the consultation and for what you might recommend in terms of investigation and possible treatment or referral. If you want to have successful consultations, you must elicit these thoughts.

Remember the little mnemonic **ICE**: **ideas, concerns and expectations**. Prompt your patient until you are sure you have a grasp of them.

CHAPTER 7

The Patient's Story of the Illness: Somatisation

Patients often worry that the doctor will not take them seriously, will think them neurotic or fussing unnecessarily. The search for a diagnosis is driven by the fear that something bad is happening and doctors share that anxiety as they try to make sense of the story that unfolds. At medical school, there is a strong emphasis on the sciences of anatomy, biochemistry, physiology and pathology, and clinical training focuses on the management of important diseases. To 'miss' a physical diagnosis is a matter for shame and sometimes recrimination.

The connection between what happens in a person's thoughts and feelings and his or her emotions and physiology is complex. Ultimately, perhaps, there is no real distinction between body and mind and my own view is that the mind is a manifestation of the complexity of the processes within the neural networks of the brain. In that sense, thoughts have physical substance, or at least are represented by subtle shifts in the structure of the brain and in the state and distribution of its atoms and electrons, quarks and forces. Our minds are our bodies and our bodies are our minds.

Accurate diagnosis of a symptom or an illness requires the clinician to look just as hard at psychological processes as at physical ones (to use the familiar divide).

Most of us will recognise that a summons to the boss for a telling-off will provoke a brisk physical response that results in a disturbance of the physiology, a shift in the motions of the body or an *e-motion*. We might reasonably characterise our emotions as physiological disturbances, hormonal and neuronal, that become manifest in our consciousness so that we perceive ourselves to be in an altered state. This alteration might be of heart rate or skin temperature, of bowel function or salivation. We connect our understanding of the stimulus to the disturbance of our steady state and we make a judgement about the phenomenon and we then say that we have a feeling.

So here then, is a chain linking a shift from the normal steady state of the body to an abstract thought. Watching a thrilling or an erotic film is a familiar experience of the mind–body link. We all know this link exists but we cannot always recognise it when it happens in a less obvious way.

Consider a child with a phobia. Perhaps she has had a frightening experience with a dog and she has developed a pervasive fear of being exposed to anything to do with dogs. She may begin to avoid certain activities because she knows her route will increase the risk of a canine encounter. Her distress increases as the fear takes hold and eventually she may be unable to leave the safety of the house without intense emotional disturbance. When presented to the doctor, such a story is relatively easily elicited and the diagnosis is clear. Treatment with cognitive behavioural therapy is usually effective. The therapist encourages her patient to have a *thought about the thought*, thus breaking the tyrannical connection between the stimulus and the immediate physical reaction and consequent reflexic avoidance behaviour. Once the child has learned the technique, she can take control of the process and once again regain her composure and the steady state is restored.

In this example it is clear enough that there is a psychological component to the physiological disturbance that the child has experienced. Patients who present symptoms for which the doctor cannot identify any underlying disease will often present cues that they themselves recognise that there is a link to psychological or emotional issues. Doctors may be very reluctant to respond to these cues, perhaps fearing the missed disease or even that they may become overwhelmed by the patient's emotional needs.[24] The limited amount of time available in primary care makes it hard for general practitioners to do justice to some patients' emotional problems. Instead, the doctor may focus upon the somatic issues, emphasising negative findings at physical examination or negative test results. This may have the paradoxical effect of increasing the patient's anxiety at not being taken seriously, forcing them to redouble their efforts at getting the doctor to pay attention to the reality of their symptoms. The vicious circle is complete when the doctor attempts to deal with this by referring for additional tests or opinions. There is then a contest between the authority of the doctor asserting negative findings and the authority of the patient whose suffering is incontrovertible. The consultation lacks authority because insufficient attention has been paid to the narratives about the presentation. Shared understanding eludes the doctor and the patient and both are dissatisfied and baffled.

A dangerous new phenomenon may now emerge. Because tests are not perfect, false positive results occur. If enough tests are ordered, misleading results accumulate and a spurious pattern may appear. Some tests, such as cardiac catheterisation, are themselves intrinsically risky and serious injury may be a direct result. If a false diagnosis is made, treatments will be recommended that may themselves have side effects. Now additional symptoms will be added to the original complaint and the picture may become hopelessly confused. If the patient is unfortunate enough to develop significant pathology while all this is going on, it will be especially difficult to make a diagnosis.

How then is the doctor to see through the difficulties that such patients present?

The approach to the consultation suggested in this book may go some way to helping. It is crucial to allow the patient to tell his or her story in as natural a way as possible. The doctor should encourage the retelling after the rehearsed story is finished so that the little details that help to place an illness in the context of that patient's whole life can emerge. The doctor must learn the patient's language and philosophy and establish the patient's ideas, concerns and expectations. Only then can validation of the patient's experience, explanation and effective management strategies arise from a consultation with real authority over the predicament.

Somatisation disorder can become a persistent and pervasive pattern in a person's life and it helps to see the current consultation in the light of those that have gone before. The harm done to the patient by earlier failures to respond to the patient's cues may have sealed the patient's fate. The patterns may be so entrenched that they are impenetrable. Success then is measured by at least doing no more harm.

There are strict diagnostic criteria for somatisation disorder. There are relatively few patients on any GP's list who meet all the conditions for the diagnosis to be made, but there will be very many more who exhibit some features and for whom this approach will be effective.

Box 9

Diagnostic Criteria for Somatisation Disorder
To qualify for the diagnosis a patient must satisfy all of the following criteria.
1. A history of many physical complaints beginning before the age of 30 and which occur over a period of several years.
2. • Four pain symptoms
    • Two gastrointestinal symptoms
    • One sexual symptom.
3. Either no diagnosis after investigation or physical complaints out of proportion to the diagnosis.
4. Symptoms are not intentionally produced or feigned.

Rule One in Torben Bendix's essay on therapeutic dialogue with anxious patients is 'situations, not symptoms'.[25]

Box 10

Rule One: Situations, Not Symptoms[26]
When neurotic symptoms appear in a patient they do so when he is in particular situations. He does not realise it, nor do you, but both of you may come to do so.

Not through your continuing to ask questions about symptoms.

Nor by your continued subjecting him to investigation for things he does not suffer from at all.

But by asking him, for example, 'Tell me about the last time you had an attack of giddiness. Where were you?' Then the patient may start talking, and it is your task to make sure that he continues until his description has revealed the situation with crystal clarity . . ..

It is not sufficient to learn that the symptoms came on while the patient watched television. You need to know what he saw on television and what happened in the room.

In summary. Try for five minutes not to use the questions 'how?' and 'why?' but try instead the words 'when ?' and 'where?'

The great gift that general practice can offer such patients is continuity. Understanding the risks of making the patient worse by failing to validate their experience or acknowledge their expertise in their own body helps the doctor to quieten the medical school-induced fear of 'missing the diagnosis'. A deal that I often agree with my somatising patients is that I will listen carefully to every presentation and consider them thoroughly. I will weigh up everything that I elicit and *together* we will make a judgement about the next step. I make it clear that the decision will be a joint responsibility and that I will see the patient again at a planned and pre-agreed interval to re-evaluate the condition.

In the long term it is possible to reduce the anxiety experienced by the patient and the costs incurred by obsessive investigation of symptoms. As the relationship between the doctor and the patient matures, new opportunities emerge for understanding of the underlying mechanism of the patient's predicament.

Through concentration on the situations rather than the symptoms, opportunities will arise that guide the doctor towards recognition of the emotional background to the symptoms and the psychosocial factors that emerge in the course of the therapeutic dialogue. Over time both may come to recognise and accept the connection between the patient's emotional state and the symptoms that trouble him or her. As understanding and acceptance grow, the patient will appreciate the validity of the reassurance that the contract provides.

Good management of such presentations is a triumph of medicine and benefits the sufferer and the health economy.

The Doctor's Story of the Illness

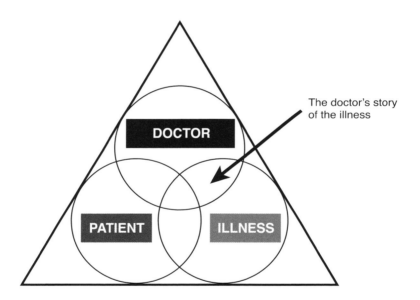

The doctor's story
of the illness

FIGURE 9 The doctor's story of the illness

He knew the cause of every maladye,
Were it of hoote or coold or moiste, or drye,
And where engendred and of what humour;
He was a verray parfit practisour.

Geoffrey Chaucer, regarding 'a Doctour of Phisike',
The Canterbury Tales (1387)[27]

BEING AN EXPERT

Now at last you can put some of your hard-earned professional skill into action. You have paid attention and listened, you have elicited the fractal beauty of the stories and you understand the patient's ideas, concerns and expectations. Now what?

Now, and only now, is it time to start *taking* a history.

One objection that students often raise when being taught about these patient-centred methods I have described here is that in ordinary life the 10-minute consultation does not provide time for the luxury of listening.

On the contrary, evidence shows that **it is precisely because time is so short that you need these techniques if you are to meet your patients' needs**. This method is much more efficient than mere sieve questions. The truth is that you will already have elicited almost all of the information you need and, indeed, you will find that large parts of your standard routine questioning can be abandoned, either because you already have the answers or because these answers would be completely irrelevant to the problem in hand. However, you may now go ahead and ask all the closed questions you need to in order to be sure of completing a safe medical history. You will find that your patient responds willingly to questioning and is relaxed and communicative with you, not least because of the trust you have earned from the first seconds of intent listening that you provided for her right at the beginning. For those wishing to learn more, examples of primary research on the effectiveness of different questioning styles come from work done in child psychiatry clinics by Rutter and Cox.[28] and there is a helpful review of the evidence for the use of open and closed questions in Silverman, Kurtz and Draper's *Skills for Communicating with Patients*.[29]

Box 11

Open and Closed Questions
Closed questions can be answered directly and briefly with just the information that was asked for. Open questions invite thought and reflection and the answers require effort on the part of the patient. Often they are not technically a question but, rather, a statement that implicitly asks for a response. Use open questions while you are trying to facilitate the storytelling process. Use closed questions to fill in the gaps in the medical history.

An example of a closed question is:
Did you have sausages for lunch today?

An example of an open question is:
Tell me about your lunch today.

You will see immediately that all you will learn from the first question is a very limited piece of information about the patient's lunch. If you are investigating an outbreak of food poisoning caused by sausages, then you will find out exactly what you need to know. If, on the other hand, you want to learn something about the patient's life, the second question will tell you much more.

Paying attention is a mark of respect when a story is being told, and there is no better way of confirming to a storyteller that you have been paying attention than by asking intelligent questions about what you have heard. It will be even more impressive for the storyteller if you are able to give a brief summary of what you have heard.

Summarising can be done in just a few phrases – perhaps confirming the chronology of the problem and the ideas, concerns and expectations you have elicited. This will prove to your patient that you have been giving him or her your undivided attention. Also, if your mind did wander at any stage, it will give your patient the chance to put you right on any details you may have become muddled about.

There is a strong probability that by now you will have started to make guesses about what is wrong and you will have determined something of the diagnostic possibilities. So now you have two more opportunities to advance your understanding of your patient and the predicament presented to you for consideration today.

The first of these opportunities lies in the physical examination. Inspection, palpation, percussion and auscultation of patients grant you the privilege of touch as part of your enquiry. There will be a rich exchange of information during the examination as you glean information from the techniques you have been taught and the patient senses your concern, compassion and respect as you go through your routine. The bond between you during the examination may well prompt some additional storytelling or re-evaluation of the narrative.

After the examination it may well be time to tell something of the doctor's story of the illness. You may wish to use what you have learned and understood so far to add some helpful background information. After all, the patient has consulted you because he or she has reached the end of his or her own resources. They have come to you for additional resource and your hard-won scientific training. Your knowledge of pharmacology, anatomy, biochemistry and physiology, of surgery and medicine and psychiatry and paediatrics are likely to have a part to play. It is your task now to add a thread or two to your patient's narrative.

Patients like doctors who explain things properly. The reason is clear enough: good explanations leave patients in charge of themselves again, and autonomy (the goal of the consultation) is enhanced. Disease is demystified for the patient and the locus of health control is shifted appropriately back towards the patient. Using what you have learned from the patient, your explanation can be pitched at the right level for him or her. It can address the very ideas, concerns and expectations that you have elicited and it can educate, motivate and inform and, above all, relieve anxiety.

Box 12

A Good Explanation
- Uses language the patient can understand
- Proceeds at the patient's pace
- Allows time for questions
- Often uses written notes and drawings
- Is tailored to fit the individual
- Uses appropriate imagery, analogy and examples
- Enhances the patient's self-esteem
- Improves the patient's ability to take responsibility for him- or herself
- Shifts the locus of health control towards the patient

A frequently used textbook on my shelf in my consulting room is *Grant's Atlas of Anatomy*.[30] It is the starting point for many brief tutorials that seek to allow patients to see something of what is inside their bodies and to begin to make connections between the story of illness and disease that they have been telling and my story of the same illnesses and diseases. When appropriate, I use a sketch pad or leaflets and pictures from the internet and from my collection that I have acquired over the years. My ear, nose and throat pictures are even laminated so that I can draw all over them while I tell the doctor's story of the illness.

The intention at this stage of the consultation is to enhance the patient's ability to make sense of what they have noticed about themselves. During your storytelling, your patient will be trying to make sense of what you are saying and trying to fit the new information that you are presenting to them into a framework that makes it intelligible.

When the process works well, there is a lot of nodding and aha-ing. The patient's understanding grows and their confidence in the power of the consultation to help them increases steadily.

Sometimes the new story appears only to add confusion. This is a very useful warning sign that the wrong tree may well be being barked up. A mismatch between the story you are telling and the story the patient has brought you will need to be examined and understood. You may need to go back to the beginning so that you can determine where you have missed something crucial in the narrative.

Do not worry that you might look clumsy or ignorant because you have got it wrong – your patient will trust you all the more if you show that not only do you listen intently but also you think very hard about what he or she is saying and that you are not prejudging the matter. 'Back to the drawing board' can be an excellent way of reaching the best solution to a problem.

CHAPTER 9

The Doctor–Patient Relationship

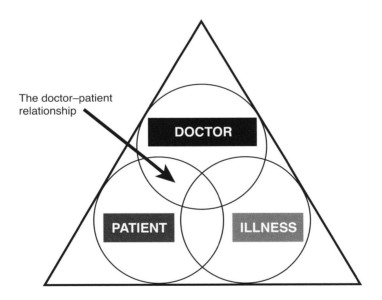

The doctor–patient relationship

FIGURE 10 The doctor–patient relationship

> *He holds him with his glittering eye –*
> *The wedding guest stood still*
> *And listens like a three year's child;*
> *The Marinere hath his will.*
>
> ST Coleridge, 'The Rime of the
> Ancyent Marinere' (1798)[31]

PAYING ATTENTION (FOR 3 SECONDS)

By the force of his will the Ancient Mariner held the attention of the wedding guest, and both became locked into the intensity of the story that unfolded.

Eliciting the narrative is the fundamental skill that underlies consultation. Some patients are as keen as the Mariner to tell their story, but others need more coaxing.

Time is of the essence, of course. Some lucky individuals have fine offices, secretaries to protect them from being disturbed, the luxury of an hour or so for the consultation and only one or two clients per day. You and I are probably different. We work in crowded, noisy places. We are constantly being interrupted. So how can you make your patient feel that this is a moment for him or her, where they have your undivided attention?

Box 13

The Present Moment

I strongly suspect that we simply happen in segments and intervals, we are composed of frames, flickering like frames of a film strip in a projector, emerging and collapsing into snake-like loops on the floor, called the just-elapsed past.

And since we live permanently convinced that the past is past, ... and the future, even the immediate future will certainly be even better and with fewer errors, and since we live permanently removed from and critical of our own past, permanently removed from and in the hope of our oncoming future **the present-time frame of several seconds is the only unconditional manifestation of our ego.**[Emphasis added]

Miroslav Holub, *The Dimension of the Present Moment: Essays*[32]

The plain truth is that to give your patient the experience of being listened to, you actually have to pay attention. Unfortunately, as the Czech poet and immunologist Miroslav Holub[33] has pointed out, humans are only designed to pay full attention in 3 second bites, but at least that is a start. Like arriving early on your first day at work in a new job to create a good impression, starting off the consultation with complete attention will reassure your patient and set the tone for what follows.

It is a rare thing, complete attention between two people. Patients notice it quickly when a doctor pays them that compliment. Attention is signalled by looking at the person, by making eye contact, by stopping doing anything else (especially with computer keyboards) and by not intruding with jokes, comments about the weather or questions.

Having created a safe and intimate space, the drama of the consultation is about to unfold. When you begin a consultation, make sure that you create this moment of stillness and attention. Often after that it is necessary to set the patient talking with a little phrase or introduction, perhaps a nod of the head or a 'How can I help you today?' The cues are recognised and the patient knows that it is their turn.

Much of the difficult work of the consultation has already been done! You have shown the patient that you are respectful of them, that you are not going to trample on their sensibilities and that you understand when to be quiet.

> *I have spread my dreams under your feet,*
> *Tread softly because you tread on my dreams.*
>
> William Butler Yeats,
> 'He Wishes for the Cloths of Heaven' (1899)[34]

Whatever the difficulties of the surroundings, you have created a space in which the two of you can operate. Emotional space is created by giving attention, regardless of what is going on around you.

The emotional space that you have defined with your attention is similar to the personal space that exists around each of us.

Box 14

Personal Space

Personal space is the area around a person that he or she regards as his or her territory.

In a doctor's waiting room with just one person in it, that person's personal space will extend for a few chairs around him. When a new person arrives and sits right next to him, he will feel uncomfortable. One would have expected him to respect the first-comer's territory and sit a couple of seats away. However, if the room becomes crowded, the area that defines personal space contracts. If there is only one empty chair left, a newcomer will sit in it without causing any discomfort to his neighbours (assuming he sits modestly, without sprawling and crowding those next to him).

On a packed London Underground train, personal space may be defined more by behaviour than proximity. If you are pressed up against someone by the crush, you know that you have to keep very still. To make a lot of fidgeting movements invades the other person's space (and invites embarrassing misunderstanding).

Box 15

Alastair, a student, entered the consulting room. He was dishevelled and downcast. He slumped in the chair. I turned to him, sat squarely facing him and looked attentively towards him, saying nothing. After a brief silence he glanced up at me and I returned his look, meeting his eye momentarily. I waited, feeling the burden he was carrying in the space between us. The empathy that this communicated elicited a deep sigh from him and he launched into his story.

WHAT IS STORYTELLING?

Most languages have a version of 'Once upon a time . . .'

> *Il était une fois . . .*
> *C'era una volta . . .*
> *Érase una vez . . .*
> *Es war einmal . . .*

There is an element of ritual and play in storytelling, which helps the listener and the storyteller to orientate themselves in relation to the culture in which the story unfolds. The same is true in the doctor's consulting room, and the doctor must do everything possible to create a setting that is conducive to storytelling. When storytelling is going well, and the listener and the teller are both active participants, there is balance, harmony and agreement.

The words we use tell us something important: History *taking*. Story*telling*. History taking is something that is done to the patient. It is an activity wholly driven by the doctor. It is a display of your ordered mind, your ability to remember a series of questions – a demonstration of your ability to dissect the patient's life to extract the information in which you are interested.

Storytelling, on the other hand, is a patient-centred activity. It is a process in which the patient has centre stage to reveal his or her experience and individuality to you. The way in which you listen will make all the difference. In 1976, Byrne and Long[35] were among the first researchers to demonstrate that serious misunderstandings occur between doctors and their patients because they did not listen to each other. Beckman and Frankel[36] in 1984 went on to show – amongst many other failings – how frequently doctors failed to allow patients sufficient time and opportunity even to finish their opening statements!

Box 16

Active Listening

- Giving the other person your undivided attention
- Letting the other person sit in silence and collect his or her thoughts if he or she needs to
- Questioning the other person tactfully and without intruding
- Trying to see the other person's point of view even if you don't agree with it
- Refraining from offering advice
- Encouraging the other person to tell the own story in his or her own words and in his or her own time

Box 17

Casual Listening

- Looking around the room or glancing at your watch while the other person is talking
- Finishing the other person's sentences for him or her and correcting his or her grammar
- Butting in to tell the person how you once had a similar problem
- Making a snap judgement based on accent, dress or appearance
- Telling the other person what you would do in his or her place
- Saying you understand before you have heard the whole story

We need now to return to the story of the relationship between the doctor and his patient. You have begun to get to the heart of the matter. You have listened to your patient's opening gambit, the rehearsed story, and you have successfully prompted them to retell the story in their own words, in much more detail and including some of the patient's own ideas, concerns and expectations, but what if things get stuck?

Patients are often very reluctant to put their own ideas, concerns and expectations into the consultation, feeling that they may be encroaching on the doctor's territory – the sacrosanct area of diagnosis and treatment. After all, if they knew what to think of the illness and what to do, they would not be there!

Torben Bendix, in his invaluable 70-page book (now sadly out of print) *The Anxious Patient*,[37] suggested seven rules for the therapeutic dialogue. They are relevant to almost every consultation you will have. We met the first rule – 'situations, not symptoms' – during the earlier consideration of somatisation.

Box 18

Adapted from Torben Bendix's Seven Rules of Thumb[38]
Rule One: **Situations, not symptoms**
Rule Two: **Repeat the patient's last words** (or possibly other words in his or her last sentence)
Rule Three: **If you don't know what to say, keep quiet**
Rule Four: **There is one, and only one, way of interrupting a pause**
Rule Five: (At this stage) **never answer questions**
Rule Six: (At this stage) **never give advice**
Rule Seven: **You must repeat and summarise**

If you are to set the patient free to expand on their story and give you the vital extra clues that will help you to understand their needs, you must devote some time and energy to the relationship between you. You must invest effort in excluding yourself from their story and not intruding.

Bendix's rules for the therapeutic dialogue will unlock your patient's reluctance and give them permission to expand their thinking without the distortion of the ideas of the expert doctor.

You may be an expert on illnesses but you cannot claim to be an expert on this patient's life. Their story has a long way to go before you can claim to have understood it.

Rule One (situations, not symptoms) was discussed earlier while dealing with somatisation. Now let's look at the remaining rules.

RULE TWO: REPEAT THE PATIENT'S LAST WORDS (OR POSSIBLY OTHER WORDS IN THE PATIENT'S LAST SENTENCE)

When your patient comes to a halt in their narrative and it appears to be your turn to speak, it is all too easy to barge in and start asking questions, lapsing into the medical model of *history taking*, rather than allowing the much richer process of *storytelling* to continue. Instead of asking a question from your 'medical sieve', such as 'How many bowel actions do you have each day?' try repeating something they have just said back to them. This will emphasise to them that not only were you paying complete attention but also you are interested in what they were saying and want to know more. You can think of it as picking up the lost thread of the narrative and handing it back to them with an encouraging gesture.

RULE THREE: IF YOU DO NOT KNOW WHAT TO SAY, KEEP QUIET

This is a hard rule to follow. It would almost be impolite under the ordinary rules of conversation, but it is important to remember that in everyday chat, people rarely employ the sort of active listening that facilitates the telling of a complete story. In chatting, the narrative thread is being handed back and forth. You are doing something quite different. You are investing in a therapeutic relationship, encouraging the unfolding of a story. So, if you do not know what to say, take a risk and say nothing at all. Maintain your attention and make sure that your patient knows you are listening carefully, still interested and just waiting for them to continue. If you find the silence unbearable, you might permit yourself an 'Mmm' or an 'Aha', but just keeping quiet is best.

Kate Fox is an anthropologist who decided to venture into darkest England to study the natives. She wrote about her work in her book *Watching the English*.[39] Her technique was to observe the strange customs of our society and postulate rules about our behaviour and attitudes. She then tested each rule with rigorous fieldwork, looking for its application and exceptions. When she was confident that she had developed a good rule that she could use to predict English behaviour, she put it to the ultimate test: she would repeatedly break the rule, in public, in as many situations as she could devise. She found this difficult to do sometimes. 'Pushing in' in a queue proved nearly impossible for her. Every fibre of her being screamed to her that to do so was wrong: she had discovered a powerful English rule. You will need to adapt the familiar rules of taking turns in conversation, however difficult that may seem, so that your patient can develop her story uninfluenced.

RULE FOUR: THERE IS ONE, AND ONLY ONE, WAY OF INTERRUPTING A PAUSE

What is a pause? There is a clear difference between your patient halting in their narrative, expecting you to speak, and a thoughtful pause. When your patient pauses, he or she may be considering, thinking, processing. This is a time of vital creativity.[40] They are making connections, assembling ideas and evaluating. Why would you ever want to interrupt such a valuable process? They will start again when they are good and ready. The creative juices are flowing but a clumsy intervention from you will dry them up instantly and perhaps irretrievably. Don't trample. If the pause goes on for a very long time, you might invite them to share some of their thoughts with you with a gentle question: **'What's in your mind at the moment?'**

Such is the power of the pause in the consultation; they should be sought and valued as early as possible. Bendix even suggests starting the consultation with an attentive pause instead of a formulaic question. Attention to all the patient's cues, verbal and physical will pay dividends and save you time.[41]

RULE FIVE: (AT THIS STAGE) NEVER ANSWER QUESTIONS

During this early stage in the consultation you are just a humble seeker after truth. You have the privilege of hearing a story unfold, told in the vernacular and freshly delivered. It would be so easy to slip into wise doctor mode, and for an expert there is nothing more seductive than being asked to be wise. I am sure that you could give a very good answer to a question asked during the early narrative, but do try to hold back. It can be difficult to recover the narrative once you have interrupted it and your undisputed genius may well inhibit your patient's storytelling and thinking.

RULE SIX: (AT THIS STAGE) NEVER GIVE ADVICE

The right to give advice has to be earned. You do not have that right just because you are a medical expert. You have not acquired the knowledge you need in order to qualify as an expert in your patient's predicament. However much you may know about their disease or illness, you do not yet know enough to offer them anything that matches their need. Once again, a premature display of your prowess will inhibit the fragile processes of discovery. Your patient may then leave at the end of the consultation without their ideas, concerns and expectations having been elicited and their needs met. You will have missed the opportunity to be a healer rather than a mere expert and your day (and theirs) will be the poorer for it.

RULE SEVEN: YOU MUST REPEAT AND SUMMARISE

As the narrative comes to an end and perhaps at key stages during the storytelling, you can encourage your patient further by repeating and summarising what you have heard. The child psychiatry clinic research mentioned earlier by Rutter and Cox.[42] showed that summarising helps patients to contribute more to the consultation. Summarising serves to reassure your patient that you have been putting your energy and talent into paying attention rather than thinking about global warming or al-Qaida. It also provides an opportunity for your patient to correct any misunderstandings that may have arisen. Bendix suggests encouraging your patient to join in the process of repeating and summarising, as this is less likely to distort the patient's priorities in favour of your own. He also prompts you to notice whether there appears to be something deliberately avoided or left out and to 'provoke yourself occasionally by thinking:

everything the patient says is true, even if it happens to mean the opposite of what it implies.'[43]

Box 19

Try Not to Say Too Much

Patient: Doctor, I've got an ache in my neck and I'd like you to prescribe a painkiller.

Dr: Aha.

Patient: Yes, it's really getting to me, especially at work.

Dr: At work?

Patient: I'm doing two people's work at present and it's weighing me down.

Dr: Mmm . . . two people's work.

Patient: Yes, I seem to get all the difficult jobs.

Dr: How does that make you feel?

Patient: It's unfair.

Dr: Yes, it must seem unfair.

Patient: (after a long pause) I don't know what I can do about it.

Dr: What would you like to do?

Patient: Tell my boss, I suppose . . .

Dr: Tell your boss?

Patient: (after another pause) But I couldn't.

Dr: You couldn't?

Patient: No.

Dr: Mmm.

Patient: Well, I have never really had the confidence.

Dr: Mmm.

Patient: Perhaps I *could* try, but what would I say?

Dr: What would you like to say?

and so on . . .

CHAPTER 10

The Three Golden Questions

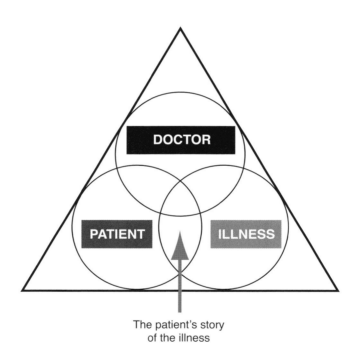

FIGURE 11 The patient's story of the illness

Seldom, very seldom does complete truth belong to any human disclosure;
seldom can it happen that something is not a little disguised, or a little
mistaken.

Jane Austen, *Emma* (1815)[44]

By now you will be close to the heart of the matter. You will have heard a rich narrative of the patient's predicament and you will understand a lot about why the consultation has happened at the exact point that it did. The story will be coherent.

It is time for you to start behaving more like a doctor. You will have been trained to ask questions. I have one more task for you before you are allowed to get on with your questions about bowel habit and bloody fluxes and all the usual doctorly business that you learned at medical school and at the surgical Grand Round.

This stage of the consultation is a good time to check that you have elicited the patient's perspective. (Having used the Bendix rules in the first part of the consultation, there is a good probability that you will have elicited most of what you need to know.) Over the years I have experimented with different forms of questions to elicit patients' ideas, concerns and expectations. I would like to offer my 'Three Golden Questions' as a suggestion for tools for you to keep in your consultation box, to be used when ideas, concerns and expectations have been difficult to elicit. You might like to learn them by heart and practise including them in your consultations, if they are needed, until they are second nature, flowing easily in your consulting style.

Box 20

The Three Golden Questions

Question 1: **When this first started, what did you put it down to, in your own mind? (Ideas)**

Question 2: **What was the last straw for you, the thing that finally decided you on coming to the doctor? (Concerns)**

Question 3: **While you were waiting for this appointment, what was the main thing that you were hoping for from this consultation? (Expectations)**

QUESTION 1

'When this first started, what did you put it down to, in your own mind?'

The purpose of this question is to clarify the patient's ideas about their illness. Notice that it is in three parts:

1. **'When this first started . . .'.** The first part of the question removes the query from the present moment. It invites the patient to think back to the origin of the problem, the time at which they are most likely to have speculated on the cause of their problem. It removes them back to a time when the

doctor was not present. It might be embarrassing for the patient to present their own diagnosis when they are in the unequal power setting of the consultation. The patient may be very diffident and cautious about presenting their own humble ideas in the august presence of the 'mighty expert'. Indeed, patients often expect doctors to be put out at having a diagnosis suggested to them.

2. '. . . **what did you put it down to . . .?'** The second part asks explicitly for a report of the connections that the patient made before coming to the doctor. Note that it does not ask the patient what the diagnosis is, or what is wrong – that sort of question invariably leads to the patient anxiously joking: 'Well, that's what I've come to find out from you, doctor!' The patient will quite naturally lose confidence in you if you appear to be floundering at this stage and desperately asking them for help. The words used here put the patient at ease and invite them to give information about their understanding of disease process and causation.

3. '. . . **in your own mind?'** The last part of this question invites the expression of fears and anxieties.

Box 21

Case History (Question 1)
A patient came to me with deteriorating aching in her jaw. Her initial story gave no clue as to the diagnosis, but she seemed very worried. I asked her what she had put it down to when it first started. She looked embarrassed and said she knew it was silly . . . but she was worried because a friend had had a salivary gland cancer. After examining her carefully it was clear she was grinding her teeth in her sleep. She was able to stop grinding her teeth with the help of a shield and she was relieved of her fear of cancer.

This question is an explicit offer to pay attention to the most private connections the patient has made at a time when they were first facing the issues raised by their illness. 'In your own mind' is readily understood by patients to be an invitation to confess their thoughts without fear of them being dismissed as stupid or irrational. The patient will have the confidence to express these difficult thoughts because the first two parts of the question remove them from the here and now. This form of question may allow patients to say things like 'Well, at first I was worried it might be meningitis/a brain tumour/cancer . . . but then I realised . . .' Patients can stand aside from their fears for a moment, making it tolerable to bring them into the consultation.

Listen with all your might to the answer to this question. It can give you the strongest possible clues as to what is needed to help your patient. It will give you essential diagnostic and contextual information and will reveal much to you about your patient's predicament.

The language the patient uses to answer your question also tells you how to approach your patient's problem and helps you define the **meaning** of the illness for the patient.

A supplementary question may be needed if the patient's history is a long one, to keep things on the straight and narrow. I ask the patient: **'And as time went on, what else did you say to yourself about it all?'**

Again in three parts, the question may be broken down as follows.

1. **'As time went on . . .'.** Just as before, the supplementary question keeps the context of the question firmly outside the here and now for the moment, permitting unembarrassed expression of the patient's fears.
2. **'. . . what else did you say to yourself . . .?'** This part of the supplementary question keeps it personal, internal, speculative and private.
3. **'. . . about it all?'** This ending to the question keeps it as general as possible, allowing the patient to expand his or her story.

After you have heard the patient out in the answers to the first question you may still be left wondering exactly **why they have consulted now** in the course of their illness or problem.

You may feel there is a missing link, the final impetus to seeing the doctor seems to be missing. On to the second question . . .

QUESTION 2

> **'What was the last straw for you, the thing that finally decided you on coming to the doctor?'**

This question is about the patient's concerns and invites them to tell you more about their thoughts on the effects of the problem on their life. It frequently elicits stories about the patient's relationships with work or family. Often someone else (with his or her own set of anxieties and problems) has 'told' the patient to consult. *If you do not elicit the ideas, concerns and expectations of this other person, you may still miss the meaning of the consultation and leave the patient and his or her family unsatisfied.*

Let us once again take each part of the question separately.

1. **'What was the last straw . . .?'** The question opens with recognition that there is a threshold that is crossed when an appointment is sought. You either do or do not reach for the phone. What makes the crucial difference?

The answer to this question may well turn out to be the key to the reason for the consultation.

2. '. . . **for you** . . .?' In the end, everything acts through the patient in front of you. You have to deal with their unique problems and reactions to them. This keeps it personal.

3. '. . . **the thing that finally decided you** . . .?' In general practice we call ourselves primary care but we should be clear that for most people, seeing a doctor is a last resort. It means that they have exhausted their self-help strategies and their belief in spontaneous resolution of the problem.

4. '. . . **to make this appointment?**' Some patients will respond to this part of the question by explaining why they are seeing you in particular, rather than another professional in your team and sometimes, it may elicit dissatisfaction with the appointment system and complaints about delays and lack of availability. Negative feelings like this are never comfortable to hear, but at least now they have been expressed rather than secretly subverting the consultation.

Box 22

Case History (Question 2)
After listening carefully to a patient describe his tension headaches and after trying to elicit his ideas, concerns and expectations, I still had no clear idea of why he had presented. I asked him what had been the last straw, why he had finally decided to consult. He told me that his wife had finally lost patience with him and his constant symptoms and had thrown an ashtray, breaking the glass cabinet that housed his collection of lead soldiers. This revelation led to an exploration of the marital problems that underlay his headache.

Having used the first two questions, you are likely to have established the ideas and concerns that led your patient to consult. The final golden question helps to elicit the patient's expectations.

QUESTION 3

'**While you were waiting for this appointment, what was the main thing that you were hoping for from this consultation?**'

If you do not establish the nature of the patient's expectations, the consultation can go horribly wrong, even after a promising start. Let's look at this question in more detail.

1. **'While you were waiting for this appointment . . .'** As with the first two questions, it is very important to get the patient out of the consulting room in their imagination, and back to a time when they were comfortably removed from the eye of the expert.

2. **'. . . what was the main thing . . .?'** This gets to the heart of the matter. It invites the patient to prioritise and helps to ensure that you do not miss the central thing that the patient wants from their contact with you, giving them permission to ask directly for exactly what he or she wants.

3. **'. . . you were hoping for from this consultation?'** It is always important to remember that patients often feel embarrassed, disempowered and constrained while they are in the expert's territory. They are inclined to become passive and lose individuality, conforming to your authority and direction. This part of the question gently reminds them that their expectations are respected and actively sought by you and it asks the patient to remember that they have formed a hope or a plan that includes the input expected from you.

Box 23

Case History (Question 3)

A man of 35 consulted me about his recurrent depression. He told me that he had had episodes since his early teens and that he had learned to expect them to follow after every major life event: graduation, marriage, the birth of his children, job changes and so on. He had managed them with a combination of medications and various spells of cognitive behavioural therapy. Towards the end of the consultation, I was still not sure why he had consulted (despite having used my first two Golden Questions). I tried the third one. 'While you were waiting for this appointment, what was the main thing that you were hoping for from this consultation?'

His eyes filled with tears. He said haltingly, 'I wanted my father to approve of me.'

The patient was seeing me, the doctor, as an authority figure, cast in the role of his father. He had never had approval from his own father and wanted validation. I was able to assure him that his quest was entirely normal and wholly understandable. I helped him to find a therapist whom he trusted to work with on this and his depression resolved.

STAYING OUT OF TROUBLE

The foundation of successful consulting is respect for the individual. If you do not respect your patient you are likely to do him or her harm, either maliciously or unwittingly. The Synoptic View of the consultation promotes sufficient understanding of your patient's needs and can help avoid causing harm.

Raanon Gillon (who describes himself as a hybrid GP and philosopher) is

Emeritus Professor of Medical Ethics at Imperial College London. In an article in the *BMJ*, about work by American philosophers Tom Beauchamp and James Childress,[45] he writes that in relation to medicine, 'The four prima facie principles are respect for autonomy, beneficence, non-maleficence, and justice.'[46]

1. **Autonomy.** Have you taken care to ensure that your patient is fully informed and able to participate without pressure in the decision to proceed with treatment? Have you told the truth? Are you patronising your patient or acting paternalistically?

2. **Beneficence.** Is the treatment you are proposing for the patient likely to do good? Is there evidence for this?

3. **Non-maleficence.** Is the treatment you are proposing safe and is the balance of risk in the patient's favour? First do no harm (*primum non nocere*). Are your intentions towards your patient good? Are your prejudices showing? Do you have a vested interest in your patient's illness?

4. **Justice (fair shares).** Is the treatment you are proposing fair and reasonable in relation to the society in which you live? Are others disadvantaged by the treatment?

Pride and arrogance are dangers for the medical profession and there are plenty of caricature examples in the folklore of medicine. In the sixth century Saint Benedict wrote a 'little rule for beginners'.[47] His 'rule' was so successful that it has formed the basis for communal living in monasteries and secular institutions across the world for 1500 years. Humility is not a fashionable word today. The root of the word, however, is in *humus* or 'earth', and implies having one's feet on the ground. Benedict suggests 12 steps to achieve this centredness (*see* Box 24).

Box 24

The Rule of Saint Benedict
1. Fear God
2. Don't gratify your own desires
3. Do as you are told
4. (Even when it is difficult)
5. Own up
6. Accept the drudgery that comes with the job
7. Don't imagine you are better than the rest
8. Follow the rules of your community
9. Don't talk too much
10. Don't make fun of serious things
11. If you must speak, speak briefly and reasonably
12. Don't show off

Using Gillon's four ethical tests and guided by Saint Benedict's 'little rule', you will stay safe and your patients will benefit too. Together they are a useful antidote to the perils of narcissism and arrogance that plague the medical profession.

Perhaps the most useful skill you can learn in medicine is that of knowing your limits. Some problems are beyond your competence and most are beyond your remit. General practice has the onerous duty of making a reasonable decision about everything that is presented to the doctor. Doctors like to be helpful and patients want to be helped, and it may seem like a kindness to offer help in areas where you are in fact an amateur or out of your depth, but you will not be doing your patient a service. Remember that you have expertise only in a very limited area, and that you *will* get into difficulty if you try to pretend expertise in a field where you have no authority.

Box 25

Know Your Limits!
Do not offer to:
- service your patient's light aircraft
- navigate for your patient during his or her voyage across the Pacific Ocean
- take your patient on for marriage guidance counselling.

It is essential to your patient's well-being that you make clear decisions about what has been told to you, and that you sort out what lies within your competence and what needs onward referral.

Hugh King, one of my general practice trainers, once told me: 'If it seems particularly troublesome, difficult to organise or impossible to arrange – it is probably not general practice.' In other words, you should find doing what you have been trained to do relatively straightforward. If things seem very difficult or awkward, then perhaps you are trying to do a job for which you have not been trained or for which you are not resourced.

THE SAFETY NET

It is a good idea at this point, with the patient on the point of leaving you, to spend a little time thinking some 'What if . . .?' thoughts. Consider some scenarios with your patient. For example, what if your patient becomes more unwell? What if the careful referral arrangements you have made fall apart? What if the terminally ill patient you have been working with rallies and starts to plan for the future again? Some scenarios are more likely than others, of course, but you and your patient will feel better and more secure if some of the top possibilities are dealt with. Your concern at this point demonstrates to the patient that you are thinking ahead in their interests, that you are not frightened by the uncertainties the future may hold and that you bother enough to take time to consider the unknowable.

Have you noticed how clerks in banks deal with their work? They make absolutely sure that they have done all the tasks presented by one customer before moving on to the next. They are careful to undertake all the transactions and paperwork, file the paperwork and close the drawers before they will even look you in the eye. They do not put a pile of used £20 notes on one side, telling themselves they will count that in a minute. Everything is sorted, tidied and neat. They do not rely on memory to make an entry at a later time.

Box 26

Kitchen Rules

My son Ed enjoys cooking and he has become a head chef. At home he is able to prepare and cook a four-course meal for 16 people and serve it impeccably. He can also run a commercial kitchen turning out 200 covers in a service. Managing everything from the kitchen staff to the pot wash – clearing up the kitchen after he has used every pot, pan and utensil – is an essential part of his skill and he has acquired a clear understanding that a major part of the art of cooking is clearing up as you go along.

If your work as a doctor is methodical it will help you to avoid becoming overwhelmed by the accumulation of tasks as the day's consulting progresses. If your work surface is uncluttered and your implements are in their correct places, a sense of well-being and order attends your consulting, allowing those who enter to feel confident and at ease.

CHAPTER 11

Working with Children

When an adult comes to see you, his or her consent in telling his or her story and being examined is often implicit. With children it is a different matter. Children are often reluctant visitors to the doctor and infants have no choice in the matter at all. Physical examination can seem to them to be an invasion of their privacy and personal space, and many consultations go wrong because their consent is not sought or because their autonomy is not respected.

From the earliest age it is essential to respect the personhood and individuality of children. They too have sophisticated ideas, concerns and expectations based on their experience and understanding. They will have fears and anxieties. Children are expected to do as they are told and they are often surprised and pleased and grateful when respect is shown for their dignity and autonomy. You will be rewarded with their cooperation and confidence if you seek their consent appropriately and explain adequately. Children respond to non-verbal cues from their earliest days. Good non-verbal communication is a vital component of your consultation skill.[48]

When a child is brought to you, make sure that you acknowledge his or her presence as soon as he or she comes into the consulting room. Make brief eye contact and give an open smile and then look quickly at the adult who has brought the child. Continue your smile, and welcome, because the child will be watching carefully and taking his or her cue from the adult's reaction to you. At the very beginning of the consultation introduce yourself to the child – 'Hello, Ermintrude, I'm Dr Bailey. What can I do for you today?' A brief pause will give an older child the opportunity to start speaking on his or her own account, and that should be welcomed. The history may be a little disorganised but that does not matter at all at this stage. After listening intently to this opening story, you will be able to judge whether to continue with the child directly or whether it is time to turn to the adult. You must include both, or one or the other will feel left out and you will have missed some important evidence. When the child seems to need some help with the history, bring the adult into the storytelling and get it going again with an open question such as: 'Tell me (again) how it all started . . .' Keep up eye contact with the child and show that you are listening and paying keen attention with nods and encouraging noises or expressions of sympathy for the problem being expressed.

Consent for physical examination for older children is largely implicit, just as it is for adults. For preverbal infants and toddlers it is harder to elicit but no less important.

Even the smallest infants watch their parents carefully to see how they are responding. They are acutely sensitive to the emotional context of the inter-action and will share and reflect their parent's behaviour. You must gain the confidence of the parent first, using the techniques already described and then you must win over the child.

During the early part of the storytelling I may reach out and touch the child very lightly and briefly. I often touch a toe or an upper arm. During the touch, I smile at the parent. Often the child will look at the faces of the doctor and their parent to read the interaction. Smiling reassures the child and frequently elicits a mirrored smile from the parent. It is then clear to the infant that the little touch that has occurred is permitted. The touch is also perceived to be well meaning and benign, welcomed by the parent, and not at all threatening or worrying. As the history of the problem unfolds and the area of concern becomes clear, it may be appropriate to make another brief touch. For exam-ple, if the child is being presented with an ear problem, a fleeting touch on the earlobe accompanied by another smile will be helpful later. Infants under a year old are fascinated by facial expression and, in particular, movement of the mouth, lips and tongue. You can get rapt attention from an infant by let-ting him or her see your tongue move on your lips, often rewarding you with the delight of a smile.

Next, explain to the parent about the examination you are going to per-form. Tell the parent what you want to do, how much undressing is required and how to hold the infant for examination. Make sure that you continue to have an open, confident expression on your face and maintain eye contact from time to time with the infant, with reassuring smiles passing between you and the parent. Now you can touch a little longer. I hold the infant's earlobe for a second or two if I am going to perform an ear, nose and throat examina-tion, and then put my finger over the external auditory meatus and rub it for a moment. Only then do I pick up the auriscope and hold it gently to the child's ear. By this time, you will usually have full consent for the examination and the infant will be placid and cooperative while you gather the evidence you need for the next stage. Similar techniques work for other examinations. It is always helpful to sign to a child what it is you are about to do. Consider how worrying it might seem when you reach to feel a child's neck nodes, suddenly and without warning. Routine and second nature to the doctor, it can seem very threatening and odd to an infant. When I am about to examine a child's neck, I show the child what I am about to do on myself briefly, touching my own neck and rubbing under my ears. Now the infant has some idea of what is going to happen, and, once again, because the parent has witnessed this and is unperturbed, the infant will consent readily and without complaint. A stethoscope can be another source of anxiety for an infant. If I am going to perform a chest examination, I offer the end of the stethoscope to the child to hold while I explain what I am going to do. Making a play of warming up the stethoscope and testing its temperature on my cheek also helps. I touch the child briefly where I am going to use the stethoscope to listen and again I exchange smiles with the parent so that the infant can witness the permission. Often I cover the stethoscope with my other hand while I listen so that it is out of sight. Nine times out of ten, the infant is completely untroubled by what I am doing and the examination can proceed without difficulty or unwanted noise.

Box 27

The Healing Touch

On holiday, I once got a fish bone stuck in my throat. I was an ear, nose and throat houseman at the time, and I was filled with apprehension about the ordeal I might face in having the fish bone removed. I went to the casualty department of the hospital near my hotel. A new ear, nose and throat house officer had just taken up the post. He was nonplussed by the fact I was a doctor and an ear, nose and throat house officer too. He was not familiar with the instruments he had to use and his hands shook. After a while spent fumbling, he called his registrar. She arrived, had evident expertise with all the instruments, was full of confidence and got on with the job. The contrast between the junior and the senior doctor was so striking. Competence and ability shone from her and I relaxed and cooperated. The bone was removed with direct laryngoscopy under local anaesthetic and my holiday could resume.

Confident touch is a very reassuring and healing experience for patients of all ages. Dithering is always worrying. Deft, economical movements with clear signposting and instructions, clear consent and methodical execution of techniques inspire trust and cooperation. Calm, confident examination of a consenting infant will contribute to the authority of your contribution to the storytelling when it comes to later explanation, diagnosis and management planning. Your retelling of the parent's story, combining your knowledge and skills, examination findings and opinion of the diagnosis with the parent's ideas, concerns and expectations will carry more weight if you are accomplished at physical examination and you have respected the autonomy of the patient through the seeking of consent and demonstration of respect for the patient's privacy.

CHAPTER 12

The Social Context of the Doctor

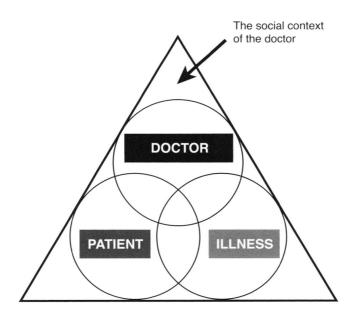

FIGURE 12 The social context of the doctor

In Chapter 2 we looked briefly at the doctor's common triad of characteristics: perfectionism, an exaggerated sense of responsibility and guilt. Now I would like to examine the social context of the doctor and suggest an additional pattern often seen in doctors that helps to explain something of medical behaviour. From reading Ovid's (43 BC–17 AD) *Metamorphoses* during your Latin classes you will remember the story of Narcissus and Echo.[49]

Box 28

Narcissus and Echo

Narcissus was a disdainful and beautiful youth. While out hunting he was seen by a nymph, Echo, who fell in love with him but she was doomed to repeat only the last words said to her. He rejected her love. Echo, ashamed, withered and died and her voice lived on only in caves. Narcissus, tired and hot, went to a fountain to drink and rest and there he fell in love with his own image, reflected in the still surface of the water. He became transfixed by his vision and he could see nothing else. Eventually Narcissus wasted away, consumed by the hidden fire of his unknowing self-love. Where he died a lovely white and yellow flower grew.

The strong tendency doctors have for believing that they are special, set apart and deserving of privilege and respect, arises from narcissism. A normal stage of infancy (usually resolved in the terrible twos, when a more mature state of relationship with the world and others evolves), narcissism can persist and influence relationships throughout adult life and careers.

Narcissists have a deep fear of discovery at their core, knowing that the power they assert is hollow. They seek to control and dominate, and their narcissism feeds their ego with beliefs of omnipotence and of being beyond the normal rules and boundaries of society.

If the helping profession's triad of perfectionism, exaggerated responsibility and guilt is combined with the narcissistic personality, the doctor who has these traits may come to believe that he or she can meet all the anxious needs of the sick and the suffering seeking relief from fear and the knowledge of death. Such doctors can inflict great injury on patients over whom they exert their power.

The certain knowledge of our eventual death ensures that we live our lives in the context of decline and illness or sudden demise. We regard our frailty with a mixture of beliefs that help us to make sense of our human condition. Some of these may be religious, or magical or scientific and we seek to manipulate our experience using interventions related to these beliefs. We pray to our gods, making sacrifices and bargaining with them or we use amulets and incantations, potions and elixirs to ward off evil influences. We invoke theories and remedies that seek to put off the awful day of death and push away the boundary of life.

Box 29

The Prophet (Khalil Gibran, 1923)[50]

For what is it to die but to stand naked in the wind and to melt into the sun?
And what is to cease breathing, but to free the breath from its restless tides, that it may rise and
   expand and seek God unencumbered?
Only when you drink from the river of silence shall you indeed sing.
And when you have reached the mountain top, then you shall begin to climb.
And when the earth shall claim your limbs, then shall you truly dance.

We live our lives in the flickering light of the camp fire, warmed by its glow but fearful of the shadows that lie outside its compass and of the watching eyes that glint there, beasts ready to take advantage of any who stray.

We contain the anxiety that accompanies the certainty of death with difficulty, and we seek to reduce our worries using the art and science of medicine. Society therefore wishes to imbue its medical professionals with special qualities, including knowledge, wisdom and understanding. We go further, even wanting our doctors to be omniscient, unerring, prescient and infallible.

Given these compatible neuroses, the doctor's desire to be in control and the patient's desire to have certainty and relief from fear, it is unsurprising that expectations on both parts will be disappointed.

Doctors, their patients and society as a whole reflect the consequences of unrealistic expectations. Fear, power, control and omniscience are all apparent in stories about medicine. There is a strong parallel with the virgin/whore perception of women. Open any newspaper and you will readily find examples of virgins and whores, and doctors as both saints and sinners.

Box 30

Medical Myths

Emergency – Ward 10	*CSI: Crime Scene Investigation*
Dr Drake Ramoray	*Doc Martin*
Dr Kildare	Harold Shipman
Doctor Who	Dr. No
ER	*Strange Case of Dr Jekyll and Mr Hyde*
Extreme Makeover	Dr Frankenstein
Casualty	*M*A*S*H*
Doctor in the House	Dr Crippen

Dr Spock	*The Tragical History of the Life and Death of*
The Citadel	*Doctor Faustus*
Dr Christiaan Barnard	*Madame Bovary*
Dr. Finlay's Casebook	Dr Josef Mengele
House, M.D.	*Nip/Tuck*

Well aware of such dangers, society and the profession itself expects a high moral tone to be set by its doctors. The Hippocratic oath and its successor, the Declaration of Geneva, reflect these expectations.

Box 31

Declaration of Geneva (World Medical Association)[51]
At the time of being admitted as a member of the medical profession:
- I solemnly pledge to consecrate my life to the service of humanity;
- I will give to my teachers the respect and gratitude that is their due;
- I will practise my profession with conscience and dignity;
- The health of my patient will be my first consideration;
- I will respect the secrets that are confided in me, even after the patient has died;
- I will maintain by all the means in my power, the honour and the noble traditions of the medical profession;
- My colleagues will be my sisters and brothers;
- I will not permit considerations of age, disease or disability, creed, ethnic origin, gender, nationality, political affiliation, race, sexual orientation, social standing or any other factor to intervene between my duty and my patient;
- I will maintain the utmost respect for human life;
- I will not use my medical knowledge to violate human rights and civil liberties, even under threat;
- I make these promises solemnly, freely and upon my honour.

When the stakes are higher – for example, when surgery is needed – our investment in our belief in our doctors becomes greater. If the organ being operated on is of critical importance – for example, the heart or the brain – our fantasy about the surgeon grows accordingly and we regard cardiac surgeons and neurosurgeons with special respect, as if their dexterity and courage and understanding were of a different order from that of the ear, nose and throat surgeon or the urologist.

Patients want to be known by their doctors; they want their physicians to understand their predicament as a whole. They seek a holistic approach that regards them as unique individuals and they want solutions tailored to their particular needs and circumstances. These requirements flow in part from the belief that someone who knows everything about them will have a better chance of making the right diagnosis and curing them of their ills.

My firm belief is that the goal of medicine is to seek the greatest autonomy possible for each patient. It is the duty of clinicians to understand and contend with the mechanisms that tempt them to believe in their own superiority. It is the task of the clinician to help patients towards self-determination.

How can the clinician hold all this in mind? The Synoptic View of the consultation can help the clinician to maintain objectivity to allow him or her to meet the patient's needs at the deepest level achievable within the constraints of the consultation.

CHAPTER 13

The Social Context of the Illness

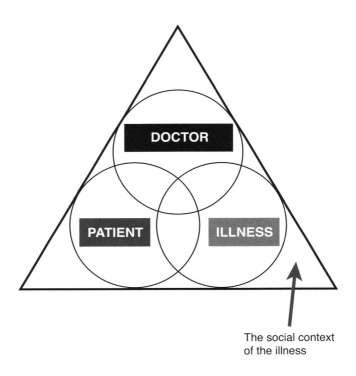

The social context
of the illness

FIGURE 13 The social context of the illness

As we have seen, the consultation does not occur in a social vacuum. Not only are the patient and doctor constrained and influenced by the social context but also diseases themselves are different in different settings and at different times in history.

In historical times it has been infectious diseases that have most exercised the concern of patients and their physicians. The terror of the spread of contagion has been a factor in society since records began. The fear of leprosy is evident within biblical stories and unfortunate sufferers became social outcasts. Plague ravaged the population of Europe in the Middle Ages, turning whole communities into ghost towns. Consumption was a constant fear and the certain knowledge of ultimate demise (often through fatal haemorrhage) that came with the appearance of blood-stained sputum haunted many families. Measles, diphtheria, polio, smallpox, typhus and sepsis after penetrating injury all took a dreadful toll of lives from infancy onward. In the decades since the introduction of antibiotics and immunisation, people have begun to forget the power of microorganisms. The emergence of HIV, Creutzfeldt–Jakob disease, severe acute respiratory syndrome and bird flu has come as a timely reminder that the antibiotic era was just a temporary advantage gained in the long struggle between mankind and infectious diseases.

The social (encompassing the geographical and historical) context of the illness will profoundly affect the consultation and the subsequent behaviours of the doctor and the patient. A disease such as malaria, which may be an inconvenience in a Fenland teaching hospital in East Anglia, may be a death sentence to a child whose parents have died from HIV and who is destitute and alone in Sierra Leone.

Cecil Helman's folk model of the consultation invited the clinician to consider the questions that are likely to be exercising the patient who is confronted by an illness.[52]

Box 32

Folk Questions about Illness
1. What has happened?
2. Why has it happened?
3. Why to me?
4. Why now?
5. What would happen if nothing were done about it?
6. What should I do about it?

The answers that the patient will have come up with and the answers that the doctor might offer to the same questions will all be influenced by the social setting in which the illness exists.

Consider the case of a woman of 50 who has type 2 diabetes and who suffers a myocardial infarction. In a society that offers care that is free at the point of use, paid for from central taxation and which values continuity of care and preventive medicine, the answers might run as shown in Box 33.

Box 33

Type 2 Diabetes and Renal Failure: The Folk Questions for a National Health Service Patient

1. **What has happened?** My kidneys have stopped working properly.
2. **Why has it happened?** Because the disease process was stronger than the medicines I was taking since I first diagnosed.
3. **Why to me?** No particular reason. It's bad luck and the odds were stacked against me.
4. **Why now?** I guess it just caught up with me.
5. **What would happen if nothing were done about it?** I will be poisoned by wastes in my blood and die.
6. **What should I do about it?** I will see my GP and specialist and get advice on dialysis, drugs and possible transplant surgery.

Living in the UK with the luxury of the National Health Service since 1948, the population has largely forgotten the value of 'free at the point of use'. Societies used to '*fee* at the point of use' value their medical services very differently.

JM Barrie's *Peter Pan*[53] was published in 1911. George Darling, father of the newborn Wendy Darling (who was to play mother to the Lost Boys in Peter Pan), knew about the worry that illness brought when medicine had to be paid for. He and his wife debated the cost of illnesses and whether they could afford to keep their daughter or whether she would have to be sent back.

Box 34

Peter Pan (George Darling Worries about the Cost of Illnesses)

'Remember Mumps,' he warned her almost threateningly, and off he went again. 'Mumps one pound, that is what I have put down, but I dare say it will be more like thirty shillings – don't speak – measles one five, German measles half a guinea, makes two fifteen six – don't waggle your finger – whooping-cough, say fifteen shillings' – and so it went, and it added up differently each time.[54]

The answers to Helman's folk model questions might look very different for an uninsured woman with the same problem but living in a fee-for-service system.

Box 35

Type 2 Diabetes and Renal Failure: The Folk Questions for an Uninsured
Patient in the United States

1. **What has happened?** My kidneys have stopped working properly.
2. **Why has it happened?** Because my diabetes is poorly controlled.
3. **Why to me?** Because I have never had anyone take any interest in my health and I have never had any checks or preventive treatment.
4. **Why now?** Something was bound to happen sooner or later, poor people die younger.
5. **What would happen if nothing were done about it?** I will be poisoned by wastes in my blood and die.
6. **What should I do about it?** There is nothing much I can do – I can't afford the medicines and there is no way I will get into a dialysis programme.

Social class is another major determinant of the effect of disease. This was recognised as self-evident and regarded as part of the normal social order throughout history. The Black Report[55] was commissioned by the UK government to examine the issue, but its socialist and re-distributive recommendations were not to the taste of the administration of the day and under the premiership of Margaret Thatcher it was never properly published. A few copies were given to the press on an August bank holiday in 1980. Its findings, however, have become the cornerstone of every discussion of the effect of social class on morbidity and mortality since then. Many of the far-sighted recommendations still await implementation.

Box 36

Broadly speaking, the evidence suggests that working-class people make more use of GP services for themselves (though not for their children) than do middle-class people, but that they may receive less good care.

Recommendation 7

Resources within the National Health Service and the Personal Social Services should be shifted more sharply than so far accomplished towards community care particularly towards ante-natal, postnatal and child health services, and home help and nursing services for disabled people. We see this as an important part of a strategy to break the links between social class or poverty and health.

Department of Health and Social Security, The Black Report[56]

Fashion is a further factor in the social context of disease. In George Bernard Shaw's play *The Doctor's Dilemma* (1906), Cutler Walpole, a society surgeon, has developed a cure-all procedure in which he diagnoses an illness in the non-existent nuciform sac and offers a treatment in which he operates to remove the diseased organ for a princely sum.[57] Shaw was satirising the gullibility of the public and the greed of the medical profession. Much complementary medicine follows the same pattern today, but allopathic doctors would do well not to become too smug. The 'do not do' recommendations on the website of the National Institute for Health and Care Excellence make interesting reading.[58] In 2011, the Audit Commission estimated that Primary Care Trusts could save up to £441 million by following the guidance and abandoning ineffective treatments.[59] Who knows what vogue of the present day will be mocked as blind prejudice in the future?

A final area to consider in these brief examples of the social context of the illness is the benefit that illness status may confer upon the patient.

In childhood, a fall or a stumble, a graze or a knock, is often followed by tears. A loving parent appears in response and administers a healing kiss and a comforting hug. In the house of one of my own friends there was a special tin of confectionery for dealing with the worst such injuries: these were called bump sweets, and only the truly brave and heroic qualified for these.

A sick person seeking the role of invalid may consult the doctor to gain the sanction and authority of the doctor in the form of a signed certificate of incapacity for work. Such an individual is then relieved of the responsibility for earning a living for him- or herself for the specified period and if it is extended indefinitely, forever. This is a very special power conferred upon the doctor and many consultations take place within this social context of illness.

A patient may experience primary gain when he or she is given a diagnosis of an illness that explains why the patient has been unable to perform a task or role that he or she had been attempting. For example, a labourer who is developing heart failure may feel guilty that he cannot work as hard and as fast as he used to but he is somewhat relieved when a diagnosis is made, as he now realises there is a reason for it, and it is not his 'fault'.

Secondary gain relates to things that lie outside the patient. Take, for example, a person who successfully pretends a diagnosis of Alzheimer's disease to avoid prosecution in a fraud case, deliberately exaggerating or fabricating symptoms. He can be said to have made a secondary gain.

These are powerful forces, and secondary gains may also operate at an unconscious level, complicating the presentation and management of disease for the unwary clinician.

The unspoken social contract is that patients should want to get better and that doctors should heal them. When either party fails to deliver on their side of the bargain, trouble follows. Doctors may become baffled or angry (or both) with patients who prefer to abdicate their responsibilities and who prefer the role of invalid. Such patients deliberately or unconsciously thwart every attempt to make them better.

CHAPTER 14

The Social Context of the Patient

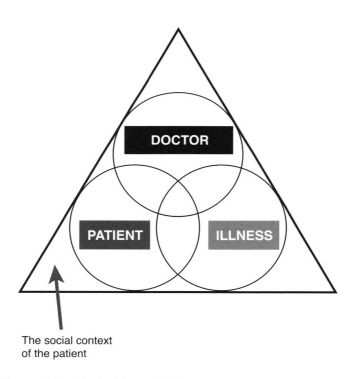

The social context
of the patient

FIGURE 14 The social context of the patient

If thou couldst, doctor, cast
The water of my land, find her disease,
And purge it to a sound and pristine health,
I would applaud thee to the very echo,
That should applaud again.

William Shakespeare, *Macbeth* (act 5, scene 3)[60]

Maps of the consultation tend to focus on the doctor and patient but commonly forget about the patient's social context. It is important to recognise that each individual is at the very centre of his or her own social web. Just as for a spider at the middle of a web, there are sensitive connections to the immediate environment. Our consciousness places us at the central point of our individual experience: how could it be otherwise? Clinicians must never forget that they are only bit-part players in the drama of their patients' lives. Clinicians have brief walk-on roles, deliver a few lines (most of which are quickly forgotten or never even heard in the first place) and then we are gone, while the rest of the action unfolds while we wait in the wings for our next cue.

So-called primary care is really more of a last resort for patients. It is only when the patient perceives that there is no other route to what he or she wants that they decide to do battle with the appointment system and seek a consultation. The social context of the patient is an important determinant of this help-seeking behaviour. It may well be that the sole reason for the attendance lies within that domain, and if you are going to have a satisfying consultation it is your responsibility to elicit this and meet their needs appropriately.

It is frequently seen in sickness behaviour that we pass responsibility for action to another person. Those we live with often take up the role of carer and it may be your patient's spouse or partner who has precipitated the attendance. This person, who is often not in the consulting room, may well be the one whose prime concern is paramount and finding out what it is that *they* are worried about can be difficult.

Consultations with more than one person at a time multiply this complexity. Consider the diagram of the Synoptic View of the consultation. Now think of it repeated for each person who enters your consulting room. Perhaps it may be a mother and father bringing a wayward teenager to you, or a stubborn, frightened, elderly man with early dementia and his worried son and daughter.

Your role as the consultation begins is to be as sensitive as possible to the influences that are not in the room. Your patient is well rehearsed in playing their character and has lived all his or her life responding to those around them. You would do well not to assume that you understand anything about them until you have some evidence.

A common scenario that illustrates some of the pitfalls for the doctor when consultation involves 'significant others' might be the tussle that sometimes occurs over certification of absence from work. The doctor's stamp of authority may be sought in order to raise the status of the patient's reason for absence. Of course, ordinary medical certificates are only appropriate if the illness has gone on longer than a week. Self-certification forms are readily available from employers and from GP reception desks, but they lack the cachet of validation, the *imprimatur*, that the physician can give to the sick role.

Box 37

My Boss Told Me I Had To Have a Note

Patient: Doctor, I had a sore throat and a cold over the weekend and I missed work on Monday. I'm better today but my manager told me I had to get a certificate.

Dr: Hm. A certificate?

Patient: Yes, doctor. She told me that I must get a note or I would be at risk of losing my job.

Dr: I am sure your manager knows that a medical certificate is not needed until the illness has caused you to miss a whole week.

Patient: Yes, but what am I going to do . . .?

Dr: Perhaps you might tell your manager that I have said that I am willing to provide a medical report but that she will need to contact me and I will charge her the normal rate for a private certificate.

Doctors can become embroiled in a tug of war between patients and employers if they collude in misuse of certification. It is important to make sure that responsibility is placed where it belongs. If the employer has a problem with sickness absence in the workforce, there is an issue to be dealt with at work. If the patient has frequent absences for minor illness, then there is an underlying issue that needs exploration. If there is an unmet medical need, then a diagnosis is required.

It is important for the clinician to remain independent and exercise intelligent thoughtfulness while the story emerges. Imagine the traps that exist when dealing with a married couple who have been sparring together for over 30 years. Each knows the other's every ploy, and every contribution is nuanced by layer upon layer of history between them. You will only earn the authority to join in through sensitive listening, and even then most of your guesses will be wrong!

The clinician needs to keep an overview (the Synoptic View) if he or she is to avoid becoming recruited as an unwilling or unknowing participant in a communication problem that lies 90% hidden, outside the consulting room.

I think of it as a sort of hovering awareness, engaged with, but not siding with, every point of view that is expressed, avoiding any premature leap to conclusion, or judgement or alliance, instead prompting storytelling and eliciting ideas, concerns and expectations for as long as necessary.

Many benefits may accrue to your patient from such an approach. He or she may gain new insight and understanding just from the exploration that you conduct with them. They may gain a new perspective simply through sharing with you the process of storytelling and reflection. Your intelligent listening may help them to hear their own story anew. You can be assured that he or she is the expert within their own life and they are likely to know most of the solutions to their unique social predicament.

CHAPTER 15

The Authority of the Consultation

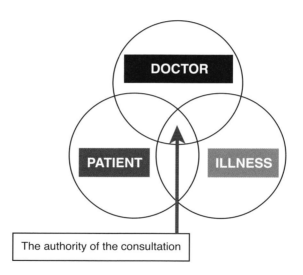

FIGURE 15 The authority of the consultation

Only connect! That was the whole of her sermon. Only connect the prose and the passion, and both will be exalted, and human love will be seen at its height. Live in fragments no longer.

EM Forster, *Howards End* (1910)[61]

Now we can turn to the heart of the matter. At the centre of the diagram of the Synoptic View of the consultation there is a domain that includes elements of all the others. This area is the goal of the consultation. I think of it as the domain of authority. Not the authority of old: the authoritarian doctor, nor yet the authority of the patient as a consumer demanding his or her rights, but the authority of understanding, respect, partnership and shared understanding that your consultation has achieved.

You have listened to your patient tell their story. You have sought their ideas, concerns and expectations. You have entered into their world of understanding and history. You have brought your own story to the discourse and you have allowed yourself to work with the flow of the stories you both bring. You have undertaken doctorly tasks such as systematic enquiry and physical examination and you have passed back to the patient something of the information you have gained, couched in terms they can readily assimilate.

You will be able to bring your experience of illness and *dis-ease* and its diagnosis, management and prognosis to bear upon the patient's predicament.

In fact, you have done all that is necessary to give this consultation authority over the issue that has been presented to you, allowing it to flow into a shared management plan that meets the true needs that have been identified.

Patients need to know the diagnosis. Although you may not be in a position to make a definitive diagnosis you should be aware of the patient's need to join with you in the search for one. There is great power in the idea of the name of an illness. Legends, myths and folk tales from many cultures recognise the power that lies in a name.

We use storytelling to bring order and give meaning to a contingent world filled with random cruelty. Knowing the names of diseases, and classifying and labelling ailments helps us to contain our fears and anxieties.

Knowing the name of the illness, the diagnosis, can retrieve seemingly impossible situations, just as the miller's daughter in the story of Rumpelstiltskin triumphs over her enemy by discovering his name.

While fairy-tale cures may rarely be possible, a diagnosis brings the hope of appropriate and authoritative management, and the consultation is, in the end, all about management. After all that has gone before, it comes down to this: what is to be done next? Once again, it is Helman's folk model of the consultation that prompts consideration of how things are going to proceed from this point.

Box 38

The Power of a Name: Rumpelstiltskin[62]
There once was a miller who was poor but who had a very beautiful daughter. One day he met the king and tried to impress him by saying that his daughter could spin straw into gold. The king put her to work in a room on her own. She was in despair. A strange little man came to her and offered to help her in return for favours. He spun the straw into gold in return for her necklace. The stakes rose as the king gave her more and

more straw to spin into gold. Eventually she promised to hand over to the little man her first child, should she become the queen. (She thought that such a thing could never happen!) The king did marry her and in a year she had her first child, and had forgotten her promise. The little man came to claim the baby. The girl was so distressed that the man said that if she could guess his name correctly he would give up his claim. She spent the days guessing many different names. She was on the point of giving up when a messenger (sent out to find unusual names) came back and told her he had seen a strange man dancing with glee and bellowing:

> 'Brew tomorrow, tomorrow bake
> After that the child I'll take,
> And sad the queen will be to lose it.
> Rumpelstiltskin is my name
> But luckily nobody knows it.'

When she confronted the little man with his true name he flew into a rage. He stamped his foot so hard that it went into the ground up to his waist. Then in his fury he took his left foot in both his hands and tore himself in two.

The doctor's story and the patient's story have combined and a new narrative can emerge. Because each has heard something of the other's story you are now ready to tell a new tale together. You know something of each other's vocabulary. As the clinician you will have heard something of the patient's *argot*, their use of the vernacular and the ways in which they use imagery. You can now contribute to the patient developing a new version of their story, retold with all their familiar themes but enriched with new ideas, themes, clues and challenges.

You can advise, based on your specialist understanding (the doctor's story of the illness) and if the patient's story of the illness is now concordant with yours, then together you have become the *authors* of a new story. It is the new story that will guide the next steps.

Shared decision making will require the exercise of considerable consulting skill. In *Skills for Communicating with Patients*, Silverman *et al.* look in detail at the evidence underpinning this element of consultation and they summarise the behaviours that the doctor should exhibit in order to achieve agreement.[63] They look at the work by Hall *et al.*[64] and Tuckett *et al.*[65] (and many others) who emphasise the paramount importance of this stage of the consultation.

Box 39

Shared Decision Making

Aims: to allow patients to understand the decision-making process; to involve patients in decision making to the level they wish; to increase patient's commitment to plans made

- **shares own thoughts:** ideas thought processes and dilemmas
- **involves patient by making suggestions** rather than directives
- **encourages patient to contribute their thoughts:** ideas, suggestions and preferences
- **negotiates a mutually acceptable plan**
- **offers choices:** encourages patient to make choices and decisions to the level they wish
- **checks with patient:** if accepts plans; if concerns have been addressed

adapted from Silverman J, Kurtz S, Draper J. *Skills for Communicating with Patients.* 3rd ed. London: Radcliffe Publishing; 2013[66]

Through all the hard work that you have done together you have a right to occupy this centre ground with your patient. You now also have a right to form a plan of management together. Any such plan will embody the shared understanding and there is a strong probability that the plan will be put into action. Both of you may have acquired tasks: for instance, it may be your role as clinician to write a prescription or make a referral or make a suggestion about a change in lifestyle. Your patient may have generated new hypotheses about his or her illness and may now be in a good position to make shifts in thinking and behaviour, use of medication, or engagement with a therapist or perhaps with another member of the family. The key thing is that the shared understanding and authority that you have both acquired enhances your patient's autonomy. The patient is now in a better position to make a *judgement* about what to do.

As a result of this approach, the patient's course of action will be a course that *they* have chosen, not one that you have imposed upon them. Doctors used to speak of compliance in relation to the behaviour of patients whom they had advised. A compliant patient was one who did as they were told, often by an authoritarian or paternalistic doctor. Later, terms such as concordance and adherence came to be used and these are much closer to the aim of the consultation that seeks the patient's autonomy. Management plans that emerge from the sort of consultation that I have described here are never authoritarian but they are usually authoritative. They are never paternalistic, but they often embody the sort of beneficent advice that a parent would offer to an adult son or daughter having taken account of a full understanding of the predicament. Also, because the management plan matches the patient's needs, it is likely to be adhered to.

What a thing it is to advise someone! It is a bold step to take and it can so easily go wrong.

Box 40

Good Advice, But . . .

In 1980 when I was first a trainee in general practice with Dr Piers Recordon in Cambridge, I saw a patient with diabetes. He was a young man who was treated with insulin. He had had diabetes for about 15 years – all through his adolescence and early adult life. He did not control his diabetes well. He had bad test results and he was beginning to show early signs of diabetic complications.

I gave him some very sound directive advice about diet, lifestyle and exercise, took his half-finished pack of cigarettes away from him and put them in the bin, and told him I wanted to see him in a fortnight. He went away and I congratulated myself on being a good doctor.

Later, when we reviewed my consultation, Piers challenged me gently, saying, 'Have you considered what it might feel like to be given advice by someone who does not know you, does not respect you and bullies you out of your cigarettes?'

The better you understand each other the more authority your shared management plan will have. It will not be your authority over the patient; rather, it will be the patient as author of his or her own life and from this will flow agreement over the chosen course of action, a prescription for a medication, referral to a specialist, a lifestyle change or waiting to see what happens.

Adherence to the plan flows naturally from the way it is created and reflects the way you have:

- honoured the past
- shared the present
- anticipated the future.

In a satisfying consultation the patient goes away agreeing with the doctor that they got what was needed. How often does this happen in reality? A study of misunderstandings about GP prescribing explored this further. The misunderstandings were all associated with a lack of patient participation in the consultation and were often based on inaccurate guesses and assumptions on the part of both the doctor and the patient.

Box 41

Categories of Misunderstanding in Relation to Prescribing[67]
Patient Information Unknown to Doctor
- Patient does not mention previous side effects
- Doctor unaware of patient's views about antibiotics
- Doctor has inaccurate perception of what patient wants: for example, assumes that patient wants prescription when they do not and vice versa
- Doctor unaware of patient's use of alternative or over-the-counter drugs
- Doctor unaware that the patient has changed the dose

Doctor Information Unknown to Patient
- Patient does not understand drug action: for example, patient thinks a steroid inhaler prevents bronchitis
- Patient wants information and doctor does not realise this or thinks that patient does not need to know or will not understand

Conflicting Information Given
- Patient confused by conflicting advice from hospital and GP

Disagreement about Attribution of Side Effects
- The doctor does not accept the patient's reports of side effects, as the computer erroneously indicates that the drug was prescribed only 2 days previously

Failure of Communication about Doctor's Decision
- Patient does not understand, remember or accept the diagnosis: for example, patient does not understand how the doctor can prescribe in the absence of a diagnosis

Relationship Factors
- Doctor prescribes and patient takes medicine, both just for the sake of the relationship: for example, patient takes medicine thought unnecessary by the doctor for fear that further treatment will be withheld

By using the Synoptic View of the consultation, the doctor may avoid these misunderstandings. A *BMJ* editorial summed up the importance of patient participation, looking at the different approaches to the consultation. It compared the traditional authoritarian approach, a consumerist approach and a shared approach involving joint decision-making and shared responsibility.[68]

Box 42

The Shared Approach[69]

Only in the shared approach do doctors commit themselves to an interactive relationship with patients in developing a treatment recommendation that is consistent with patient values and preferences. To enable this to happen, the doctor needs to create an open atmosphere in which patients can communicate all their agenda items. In this approach, information exchange helps the doctor to understand the patient and ensures that the patient is informed of treatment options and their risks and benefits. It also allows patients to assess whether they feel they can build a relationship of trust with their doctor.

There is an important difference between eliciting the patient's perspective and becoming absorbed by it altogether. The Synoptic View can help you to maintain an overview of the story, to retain your critical judgement and to see the problem that is presented to you in the rich perspective of the individual and the social context of the consultation. As a member of the helping profession you will be looking for ways to give your patient the help they are asking for. However, do not forget that other forces may be at work. The patient may be terrified of a particular diagnosis and very reluctant to have it discussed, seeking to divert you from your enquiry and proper management of the condition. Your responsibility is to stay vigilant, attentive and critical, accepting nothing at face value, suspending judgement until all the facts are in and developing a new narrative with the patient that embodies all that has to be considered and done.

Box 43

Don't Let Your Patient Brainwash You!

A 60-year-old woman came to my practice one morning and spoke to the senior receptionist. She told her that she had had chest pain for 24 hours. Her husband had wanted to call the out-of-hours service the previous evening but **she had convinced him that there was nothing wrong**. She told the receptionist firmly that she did not want to make a nuisance of herself and that she would attend the unbooked surgery starting in an hour's time, and that she would walk home to wait in the meantime. Despite clear standing orders about the management of chest pain, the receptionist **accepted her judgement and let her go**. The doctor on duty of triage calls rang the patient. He elicited a history of chest pain that had come on during exertion the previous day. He wanted to call an ambulance for the patient but she declined firmly and said that she would be happy to walk to the surgery for an appointment in the 'sit and wait surgery'. **The duty doctor complied with her wishes**. I saw the patient when she arrived and elicited a history of central chest pain that had come on during a long walk on the previous day and which had been bad enough to make her sweat. **She assured me that it was nothing and by the end of the consultation I was fully under her spell** and preparing to send her home after a normal ECG. However, the ECG was abnormal, suggestive of a myocardial infarction or pericarditis and I called a coronary ambulance and sent her to hospital. Four hours later, she was home again. The diagnosis of pericarditis had been confirmed and **she had successfully persuaded the hospital doctor that nothing needed to be done** and that she could be discharged.

It is rare to meet such a powerful patient, but the phenomenon of collusion in denial is lurking, ready to catch the unwary and the experienced alike.

Part Two

Consultations That Go Wrong: Using the Synoptic View as a Diagnostic Aid

INTRODUCTION

Consultations that go wrong can be as distressing for the clinician as they are for the patient. Despite our best efforts we will all sometimes fail to understand, fail to communicate and be unable to help. In my work with medical students, trainees in general practice, with colleagues and frequently in my own work I have used the Synoptic View of the consultation as a diagnostic aid. Once it becomes clearer where the problem lies, it is easier to work towards a remedy.

There are 10 domains to the Synoptic View model, and each of them has a readily understandable name. Each domain needs to be 'serviced' by the appropriate behaviour in the consultation so that information relevant to the problem is elicited.

When all the domains have been dealt with appropriately, the final central domain of 'Authority' is satisfied; the consultation has authority over the issue in question and the management plan flows from that, with the patient fully engaged.

When things go wrong, the problem can often be mapped to one particular domain that has been neglected or where the behaviours are dysfunctional.

Doctors who are the subject of complaints often present with a definite pattern of repeated conflict, deficit or failure. It is my hope that teachers and students, coaches and mentors, the General Medical Council and other regulatory bodies could use this model to identify the area of difficulty and make practical suggestions of what to do in order to remedy the problem.

Provided here is an overview of the 10 domains with examples of possible dysfunctions and their consequences. From this you will be able to see how the Synoptic View helps in making a diagnosis of the underlying problem in the dysfunctional consultation. Using the methods I have described, a consultation between the doctor and his or her mentor can gain authority over the problem. The management plan that emerges has a strong chance of engaging the doctor and resolving the dysfunction.

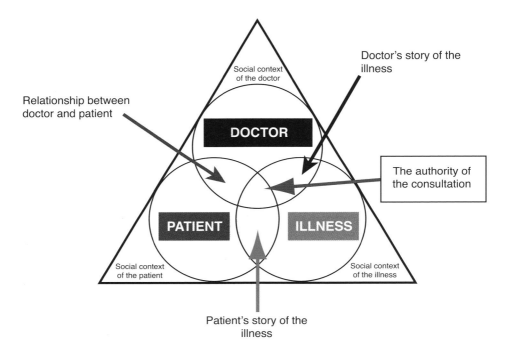

FIGURE 16 The Synoptic View of the consultation

Domain	Dysfunction	Consequence
The doctor	Burned out	Cynical and bored, the doctor becomes peremptory and disengaged
The patient	Lacking in self-confidence	Diffident and nervous, the patient finds it almost impossible to admit to having ideas, concerns and expectations that need to be taken into account
The illness	Atypical presentation of a common condition	The doctor may jump to the wrong conclusion, leading to inappropriate investigation, referral and treatments, with adverse consequences
The patient's story of the illness	Disorganised and distracted	The patient's story may lack coherence, fail to follow a timeline, be remembered inaccurately and be very difficult to follow
The doctor's story of the illness	Arrogant expertise	The doctor may be so pleased with his specialist knowledge that his main concern is to demonstrate his superior knowledge and miss the real concerns of the patient
The relationship between the doctor and the patient	The patient who is a frequent attender	The doctor may become complacent with a history of repeated attendance with minor symptoms and miss the 'red flag' of major disease
The social context of the doctor	Doctors working in target-driven units, besieged by financial imperatives	Health workers may become callous and indifferent to patient suffering and serious deficits in care may follow
The social context of the patient	Adverse history within the family of illness in the past	Unless elicited, the family's experience of illness may colour every aspect of the consultation and prevent engagement with a chosen management plan
The social context of the illness	Stigmatising illness	HIV infection in our time, cancer in the recent past and tuberculosis in the more distant past were all 'unmentionable'
The authority of the consultation	Derives from all the other domains being satisfied	When the consultation has given appropriate attention to each of the nine domains, the tenth, the centre domain, acquires authority over the predicament
When done well, the right management ensues
When done inadequately, the wrong plan emerges or the patient rejects the plan as not meeting his or her real needs

CHAPTER 16

Dysfunction: The Doctor

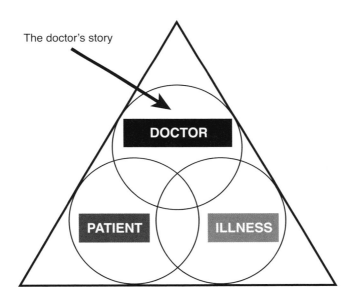

The doctor's story

FIGURE 17 The doctor

Doctors are attracted to a career in medicine for a wide variety of reasons. These reasons may change and mature as they progress from medical school through training posts and onwards to substantive roles in general practice or in specialties. The path is rarely smooth. Early hopes and aspirations may not be fulfilled, and many become exhausted by the demands of the profession. Doctors have a propensity for self-harm, which may take many forms. These may be culturally acceptable, manifesting as perfectionism and an exaggerated sense of responsibility, or they may get the doctor into trouble as he or she seeks relief from inner conflict in drugs or alcohol or illicit relationships. Depression and burnout are common in doctors in the middle stages of their working lives.

Doctors, then, are as human as their patients and their problems and ills are no different. However, the doctor's task is to meet the patient in the consultation with a clear mind and with his faculties intact and at the service of the patient and the problems presented.

Clouded judgement puts patients at risk. When doctors cease to listen and become cynical or arrogant or dismissive, the patient's concerns are no longer at the centre of the interaction. Instead, the doctor's ailment distorts the consultation. The outcome may be more about the survival of the doctor than that of the patient.

Box 44

One doctor I worked with filled his surgeries with patients who were on treatment for hypertension. He would check their blood pressure and have them out of the door within 2 or 3 minutes, offering peremptory advice and a repeat prescription. After 12 patients he would go home. He was deaf to any other concern the patients might have wanted to express and not in the least interested in the management of hypertension. He was burned out and cynical and could not wait to escape from the profession.

The remedies for such doctors are as varied as the ailments that afflict them and the stories they will tell. A prerequisite for help is that the problem is recognised as lying within the doctor. The tendency for the doctor will be to deny the existence of a problem, to project it onto his patients, the system in which he works, his colleagues or the authorities. Anywhere other than where it belongs – within himself.

It has always astonished me that doctors do not have a tradition of supervision. Other helping professions have it built in to the very structure of their working lives. No psychotherapist or counsellor would consider working without supervision. Why should doctors think they alone do not need this safeguard for themselves and their patients?

Recently the General Medical Council has made it a duty of doctors to look out for impairment in their colleagues and act when it is recognised. Appraisal is well developed in general practice but remains rather patchy in hospital settings. Good appraisers may sometimes get a glimpse of the unmet needs of doctors. The additional imperative of revalidation will focus attention on the well-being of doctors. Appraisers and the officers responsible for revalidation have a duty to act to protect patients. We are likely to see increasing numbers of doctors in distress being identified. We urgently need more provision of coaching and mentorship for doctors at all stages of their careers. We should to be able to steer our colleagues towards help when we see them in need of support, and we must learn to accept that having supervision is a strength and not an admission of weakness. Seeing the doctor as integral to the consultation and not separate from it may help us to recognise the importance of the physical, emotional and mental health of the doctor.

Using the Synoptic View as an aide-memoire for the consultation reminds the doctor that he or she is as much a part of the consultation as is the illness or the patient. It prompts the doctor to remember the duty of self-care, making sure that the doctor meets his or her patients with an open and unclouded mind.

CHAPTER 17

Dysfunction: The Patient

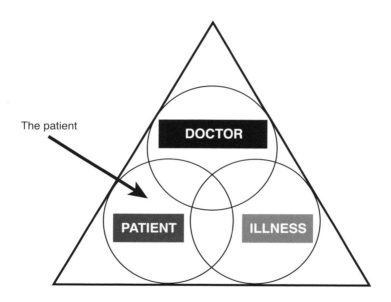

The patient

FIGURE 18 The patient

Is it ever acceptable to blame the patient when a consultation goes wrong? *'Tout comprendre, c'est tout pardonner'*, said Tolstoy. 'When you understand everything you can forgive everything.'[70] However, the doctor is not omniscient, cannot know all and cannot understand all, and I have certainly had dysfunctional consultations in which I felt I didn't stand a chance of a satisfactory outcome.

Box 45

I remember a consultation with a patient who was spoiling for a fight. I had seen her husband earlier in the week and he had told me about her controlling behaviour, jealousy, checking, aggression and argumentativeness. He was at his wits' end and wanted to separate, but wanted custody of his son who he felt had a better chance of a balanced life in his care rather than his wife's. She came to see me and the atmosphere crackled with tension from the moment she came through the door. She challenged me throughout the consultation. She wanted to know what her husband had consulted about; she wanted to determine exactly what I wrote in my medical record about her. She wanted to know if there was inaccurate third-party information about her in her husband's records. She challenged my knowledge of Caldicott principles for data control. When I was unable to quote the law she challenged my role as a senior partner and said that she was going to lodge a formal complaint of incompetence. I asked her as gently as I could whether there was anything practical that I could help her with today. In response, she demanded my General Medical Council number and then wanted an immediate appointment with a colleague instead of me. She refused to leave the consulting room until I had arranged for her to speak to the practice manager immediately. She finally left the room (to my immense relief) after a full 25 minutes.

When I had recovered my equilibrium, I reflected on what I might have done differently. I might have said something like 'I can see that you are very angry at the moment – I wonder if you would like to tell me more about it?' She did, in fact, consult me again, and I tried something like this but she became incandescent with rage and told me to stop being an amateur therapist and stick to what I knew, 'which is evidently not much', she said.

So, yes, the patient *is involved* when the consultation goes wrong. As doctors we must remember that we are bit-part players in someone else's drama. We don't have the benefit of knowledge of their life script, and if they don't want to be helped we may have to accept that our role is to take it on the chin, and keep lines of communication open unless boundaries of acceptable behaviour are crossed. Our duty is then clear, a duty to the patient, to ourselves, to our staff and to the other patients waiting for their turn with the doctor. We must defend the boundary, setting limits and exercising control and asserting our right to decline to work with someone with whom a therapeutic relationship is impossible or even dangerous. Vexatious complaint may be extremely damaging and distressing to those caught up in the machinery of investigation. Malicious patients, especially if they are highly intelligent, literate and plausible, can use well-intentioned complaint systems to terrorise a clinician who falls foul of them.

Patients as challenging as the one I have described above are fortunately very rare. However, patients with a hidden agenda are not unusual. Those seeking secondary gain – a motive that is not expressed and an intention to gain an advantage that is not declared – may hide their plot very thoroughly and deliberately subvert the doctor's honest intention to get to the heart of the matter, deal with the problems that are presented and work with the patient to resolve his or her issues. Addicts seeking drugs, malingerers seeking compensation for bogus accidents, carers exploiting elderly dependants, and parents abusing their children all pass through the consulting room at some point.

The Synoptic View of the consultation can help to identify these very difficult patients and diagnose the nature of the dysfunction. When a consultation takes you into conflict or leaves you uneasy or baffled as to the motive for the attendance, reflection using the domains set out in the model will allow you to check off what you know about the presentation as declared to you. Careful review will often show inconsistencies that will allow you to make some educated guesses. Subsequent consultations may then give you the opportunity to explore any gaps, checking and cross-referencing with what you already know.

I strongly recommend working with a colleague when attempting to understand dysfunctional consultations and especially when you suspect you have a patient presenting in this way. You need the objectivity and benefit of a disinterested third party. If both of you work systematically through the domains of the Synoptic View, you will be in a much stronger position when you next call your patient into your consulting room. You may then be able to establish the true authority of the consultation, having elicited the underlying subterfuge and motivation. Confronting and challenging these difficult situations takes courage and clarity of thought – far better to attempt this with a thoughtful colleague at your elbow and a map of the consultation that reflects the messy complexity of real life.

CHAPTER 18

Dysfunction: The Illness

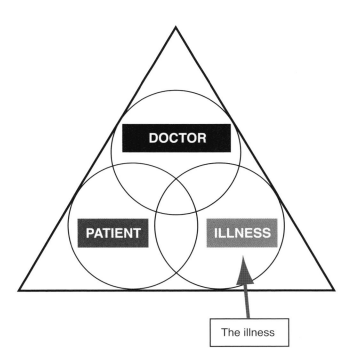

FIGURE 19 The illness

Sir William Osler said: '. . . we, the doctors, are so fallible, ever beset with the common and fatal facility of reaching conclusions from superficial observations, and constantly misled by the ease with which our minds fall into the ruts of one or two experiences'.[71] Human beings love to see patterns, which is why we enjoy looking at the shapes clouds make, why we see faces in plug sockets, and why we invent racial stereotypes. Our astonishing capacity for organisation into categories has been a driving force for the advancement of knowledge for our species, but it is all too easy to see meaning where there is none, to mistake association for cause and to diagnose before all the evidence is collected. We are inveterate classifiers. This ability has allowed us to organise the world around us to suit ourselves and to organise our thoughts to deal with the core experiences of birth, life and death. We use our insights to gain control over our lives and to thwart the processes of disease and chaos that would otherwise undermine our autonomy and our very existence.

Diseases have an independent existence, a reality, which is separate from our ability to recognise, understand and manage them. Since our trajectory through life is inexorably towards death the truth of this is inescapable. Illnesses are often spoken of as if they have characters. Our words for growths point to this, as we classify tumours into benign or malignant varieties, as if they had intention. Atherosclerosis is called a 'silent killer' and epidemics are said to 'stalk the land'.

Illness is of itself a dysfunction – a combination of disease and human response. A fundamental purpose of the consultation is the correct identification of the disease and the patient's response. When the doctor is skilful, well educated and well resourced, the disease is named and the correct diagnosis emerges from the processes of history, examination and investigations. Doctors hold their position in society because of their role in the diagnostic and treatment process. Their efforts give their patients the hope that disease can be cured, symptoms eased and disability mitigated.

When we alight upon a diagnosis, the patient who entered the room with an illness acquires a disease. This process may have a profound effect upon the future course of the patient who may undergo arduous or hazardous investigations and treatments based on our judgement. The wrong diagnosis inevitably leads to the wrong management. A premature diagnosis closes the mind to alternatives. Once we have named something, the tendency is to stop thinking about what it is, rather about how to deal with it.

Some diagnoses are just plain difficult. How many of our irritable bowel syndrome patients have coeliac disease? How many people with aches and pains have hypermobility syndrome? Which of us has not missed a patient sinking slowly into hypothyroidism? Or dementia? Who has not missed an early case of zoster or given an antacid to a woman with coronary artery disease? Who has not misjudged a terminal care prognosis by days, weeks, months or even years? Who has not missed an ovarian or a pancreatic cancer in its early stages? Who is likely to know enough about Ehlers–Danlos syndrome to distinguish between the arthrochalasia type and the progeroid form?

Our understanding of disease is partial. We do not know the cause of common diseases such as Alzheimer's disease or Crohn's disease or Parkinson's disease, and experience shows us that, as new insights emerge, new subtypes and categories emerge within ailments. Disorders recognised for centuries such as anaemia, arthritis and fever now have many subdivisions with physicians devoting their whole careers to the management of super-specialist branches of their disciplines.

It is not surprising then that misdiagnosis is the key dysfunction of the illness domain of the Synoptic View of the consultation. If the doctor neglects the patient's narrative and other pointers in the history, skimps the examination and orders the wrong investigations, the hapless patient may suffer the consequence of the wrong diagnosis. The patient is treated in the wrong category of pathology and is exposed to the harms and miseries of drugs or surgery or psychiatry to no avail.

The Synoptic View of the consultation that I have proposed can help to reduce the probability of making the wrong diagnosis. Accurate identification of the ailment is more likely if we listen to our patients' stories, and understand more about their social context. If we study their language and their own beliefs about causation and health, pay attention to their speculations and observations and respect their expertise and knowledge of their own lives and bodies. The whole purpose of the consultation is this 'getting to the heart of the matter' in order to enhance the patient's autonomy through authority over their predicament. The diagnosis needs to be couched in a biopsychosocial perspective if we are to understand what a disease means to a patient and how we are to advise them.

There is, of course, no substitute for clinical expertise. Knowledge, skills and understanding are paramount and our duty as clinicians is to learn, to practise our skills and hone our thought processes. Medicine is infinitely complex, subtle and ambiguous and we owe our patients the highest standard of care we can muster. We must keep reading, talking, sharing, challenging, experimenting, researching, puzzling and thinking.

Box 46

I once worked as a locum general practitioner for an elderly doctor whose patients had been trained to stand at the corner of his desk reciting their symptoms. As soon as this doctor could identify a matching disease he stopped the patient, wrote out a prescription and handed it over. The consultation was at an end. The patient took the prescription and left. He could easily see 30 patients an hour and when he had finished his own list he would go into the waiting room to scoop up his colleagues' patients too. He made unsolicited visits to many of his elderly patients and gave them prescriptions too. I never knew a doctor who could diagnose so many diseases in one day! His patients loved him and he was a very popular doctor, but one cannot help wondering . . .!

At the opposite end of the spectrum, there are specialists who cannot let go of their patients. They are so knowledgeable about the pathologies in which they specialise that they are inclined to think that everyone referred to them must have a rare form or an atypical presentation of a disorder in their domain of expertise. They order ever more expensive tests with increasingly equivocal results and trap patients in cycles of experimentation with treatments that can leave them exhausted and bewildered.

The remedy for these dysfunctions is an open mind. The good physician must hold his or her diagnoses as probabilities rather than truths. They must sieve and weigh the evidence as it emerges from the narratives of the consultation and the course of the illness under consideration. They must accept that they are more fallible than their anxious patients would wish them to be and they must admit their failures and mistakes. Patients respond very positively to this honesty and are more likely to forgive error and misjudgement when they can see the doctor engaging with uncertainty on their behalf.

The Synoptic View of the consultation enhances the authority of the consultation by enabling the doctor and the patient to synthesise the maximum amount of information about the problem in the shortest possible time. The right diagnosis is paramount and is more likely to emerge using the approach I have advocated. Diagnostic error is less likely to result in litigation when the doctor has been humble in the face of ambiguity and incomplete understanding.

CHAPTER 19

Dysfunction: The Patient's Story of the Illness

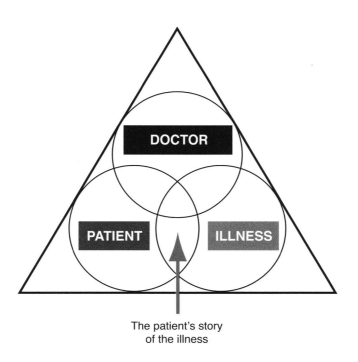

The patient's story
of the illness

FIGURE 20 The patient's story of the illness

It is often suggested that all a doctor needs to do is listen. 'The patient is telling you the diagnosis!' Would that this were literally true. Instead, the narrative that leads to the diagnosis can have many twists and turns. The Synoptic View of the consultation is an aide-memoire that reminds the doctor of the importance of eliciting the patient's story of the illness. However, if it is unchannelled, the patient's narrative may well seem to be leading nowhere. His or her story may lack coherence, fail to follow any sort of timeline, be remembered inaccurately and be very difficult to follow.

Box 47

If the consultation is to be successful in establishing authority over the patient's ailment it is essential to spend time and effort clarifying the patient's narrative.

In the absence of such clarification, the clinician will be left guessing about the reason for the patient's attendance, the nature of the problem that is being presented and the expectations that the patient has brought to the consultation. Very soon, the doctor will be addressing the wrong question, the patient will be baffled or alienated and the rapport that is essential to a cooperative management plan will be impossible. The doctor will assert authority over the predicament and diagnose, prescribe and recommend, but his wisdom and erudition will be lost on the wind. The patient will experience the consultation as unsatisfying and is likely to characterise the doctor as authoritarian, uncaring and arrogant.

A colleague of mine came to me seeking support after a particularly distressing consultation had led to a complaint about his care. He had been accused of arrogance and lack of compassion. He had been called to see a dying patient at home. The patient's husband was concerned that his elderly wife had developed intestinal obstruction because her bowels had not worked for a few days. Before the doctor had a chance to examine the patient, the husband confronted my colleague anxiously, demanding to know what should be done if the bowel were to be found to be blocked. The doctor explained that admission to hospital to resolve the problem might be required. At this, the husband became extremely agitated and accused the doctor of arrogantly dismissing the patient's wish to die peacefully at home in the company of her family. He recruited the district nurse and the patient's sister to his indignant rejection of the doctor's suggestion and all of them sent formal letters of complaint.

We looked at the Synoptic View together as we reflected on what had happened in this consultation. Slowly it became clear that the doctor had skipped a step. He had responded to the husband's anxiety, and sought to offer a management plan before he had elicited the patient's story and the social context of the patient in sufficient detail. His attempt at reassurance that he was master of the situation had had exactly the opposite effect. He had made assumptions but had wholly misjudged the situation and the wishes of the patient and her carers. He had asserted authority before he had earned it. The consultation had not reached the point where it had authority over the predicament and the management plan that the doctor had asserted was insulting to the family.

My colleague recounted other dysfunctional consultations that had led to complaints of arrogance. He had been very distressed by these, as he perceived himself to be a very caring and compassionate doctor. He had felt victimised and even a little paranoid and had become very defensive.

It was a great relief to him to discover an explanation for what was going wrong in his consultations. He decided to enrol on a consultation skills course.

The course he undertook was based on the skills of the Calgary–Cambridge observation guide.[72] Particularly relevant to him were those skills related to gathering information:

- **patient's narrative** – encourages patient to tell the story of the problem(s) from when first started to the present in own words (clarifying the reason for presenting now)
- **question style** – uses open-ended and closed questions, moves appropriately from open-ended to closed
- **listening** – listens attentively, allowing patient to complete statements without interruption; leaves space for patient to think before answering or go on after pausing
- **facilitative response** – facilitates patient's responses verbally and non-verbally (e.g. use of encouragement, silence, repetition, paraphrasing, interpretation)
- **clarification** – clarifies statements that are vague or need further amplification (e.g. 'Could you explain what you mean by light-headed?')
- **internal summary** – periodically summarises to check own understanding of what the patient has said; allows patient an opportunity to correct interpretation and provide further information
- **appropriate use of language** – uses concise, easily understood questions and comments, avoids or adequately explains jargon.

After the course, my colleague felt a burden had been lifted from him. He had a clear model for what he had to achieve and he had the tools to match the task. He has had no further complaints.

CHAPTER 20

Dysfunction: The Doctor's Story of the Illness

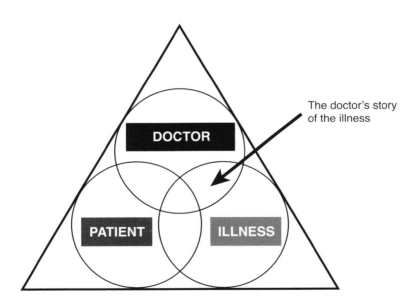

The doctor's story of the illness

FIGURE 21 The doctor's story of the illness

The human mind is designed to leap to conclusions. We process information at an astonishing rate and make guesses and judgements about what we see and hear. For instance, when we are talking together we unconsciously anticipate the next word that is coming from someone we are listening to. This helps us to understand what they are saying and fill in missing data. This is especially useful when we are in a noisy environment, when we recruit a bit of lip-reading and observations from facial expression along with our shared experience with our companions. Some people try to speak along with those they are listening to, echoing the last words of each sentence as it emerges from the speaker. One of my patients was particularly assiduous in this exercise and I found it very distracting, as I mischievously strained to avoid the expected word and insert something unguessable for my listener!

Box 48

A common dysfunction in consultation arises from the tendency to rely upon judgement by first impression. The doctor's story of the illness overtakes the patient's and dominates the consultation. The doctor may be so keen to be an expert that he or she stops listening as soon as it is 'obvious' what the patient's problem is. Arrogantly asserting control, the doctor silences the patient and begins to issue instructions and advice, prescriptions and directions.

The Synoptic View of the consultation helps to remind the physician that his or her story of the illness is just one facet of the whole, and that in order to help the patient in their unique predicament, all the domains must be respected and relevant information elicited if a helpful management plan is to emerge.

Specialisation allows expertise to be refined and knowledge of complexity to be focused on the minutiae of disease. Thank goodness for experts. I definitely want my diseases to be managed with the help of experts! I also want my ailments to be understood in the context of my own life and experiences, hopes and aspirations. A major achievement of general practice at its best is the cooperation that can be established among the patient, the general practitioner working as a physician with an overview, and with a specialist who is expert in the complexities of molecular management or surgical dexterity. The unhappy downside of specialisation is that the expert may become much more interested in the organ than the person, the enzyme rather than the entity. Such experts may come to regard all the other domains of the Synoptic View as troublesome irrelevancies rather than essential components of the struggle to make sense of illness and mortality. The caricature of the arrogant consultant striding along the ward with a retinue of followers to teach the juniors on the ward round about the 'Liver in Bed 10' still resonates. I suspect that everyone working in medicine today could still point to a colleague who fits the bill.

The Synoptic View is an antidote to this arrogance. Every domain has its own authority and taken together they can confer real authority on the output of the consultation.

CHAPTER 21

Dysfunction: The Doctor– Patient Relationship

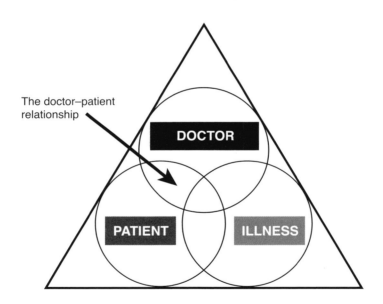

FIGURE 22 The doctor–patient relationship

One of the privileges I valued most during my 24 years as a partner in general practice was the continuity of primary care. Young people who knew me in their teens as I came into the profession grew up, formed relationships, had babies and brought them to me, confident that they were seeing someone whom they knew and trusted. I watched some of those babies grow into adults and then have their own children. Three generations of knowledge and understanding. Such relationships inform and enrich the consultation. Confidences and secrets can be revealed, hopes and fears admitted to and disease, illness and mortality confronted.

The essence of the benefit of continuity of care is the trust and understanding that flows from the time spent together. Fortunately for today's fragmented society these delicate blooms can grow very swiftly. Even during the course of a single consultation a bond can form very swiftly between the doctor and the patient. Respect for the patient's narrative, careful attention, elicitation of the patient's ideas, concerns and expectations, followed by clear exposition and explanation and careful negotiation over management can result in a patient being delighted, deeply touched, and eager to commit to working with the doctor in the future.

The shadow side of this ideal reveals itself in complex ways. The doctor–patient relationship can become dysfunctional in the infinite variety of ways that complicate all our dealings with other people. The relationship is as complicated as those of husbands, wives, sons, daughters, employers and employees – indeed, of all human connections.

Overfamiliarity can lead to complacency. This is a particular risk for the patient who is a frequent attender. The doctor and the patient fall into a pattern of behaviour in which they both act their familiar roles. Under this cloak of repetition, collusion to avoid deeper issues can occur or new diseases can emerge, hidden by the blindness of seeing only what one expects to see.

The Synoptic View, with its careful emphasis on the narrative, can help to guard against this complacency. Seeing every consultation as unique keeps at bay the tendency to dismiss complaints as the 'same old same old' and hold in focus the experience of the patient in front of one.

Box 49

Doctors can become very jealous of the care they give to their patients. They dispense their listening skills all day, dealing out compassion and understanding, empathy and reassurance and end the day overdrawn in their emotional accounts. When they get home to their loved ones, they have to gear up again to do the same at home – or not! Communication experts in the professional setting, they may well be reclusive, closed and silent with their families, burned out by the job. This is fertile territory for trouble. The doctor may seek analgesia for the soul in alcohol or through the use of drugs or through the formation of inappropriate relationships. The General Medical Council rightly regards intimate relationships with patients as highly unprofessional. The combination of a needy patient and a doctor jealous of all that understanding and nurturing they have doled out can result in a heady mixture of co-dependency that throws caution to the wind.

The broad overview of the human condition that is contained in the Synoptic View of the consultation lets the doctor see the patient as a whole. This wise supervision can protect the doctor against the formation of inappropriate relationships. It also provides a template for talking about work with colleagues, helping to focus attention on the areas of the consultation that may be neglected yet are crucial to the understanding of the patient's presentation.

As I mentioned earlier, in Chapter 16, I have long wondered at the anomaly of the absence of formal supervision for doctors. Counsellors and therapists have supervision built in to their roles as a professional necessity. Despite the seminal work of Balint and others in the last century, GPs and hospital consultants go through their whole careers with no formal attention to the personal needs, responses and reactions generated through their difficult work with patients. In my last practice we introduced a regular supervision session for the medical staff, led by a psychotherapist. In these meetings we could admit to and work on our feelings about and in response to our patients, understand them better and return to consultation with clearer perspectives and more insight. The Synoptic View allowed us to analyse our consultation dysfunctions methodically and swiftly.

CHAPTER 22

Dysfunction: The Social Context of the Doctor

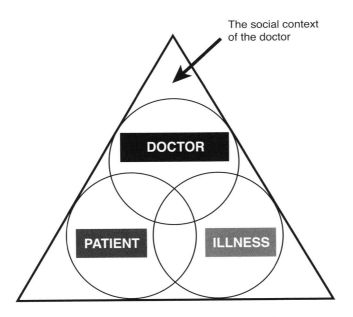

FIGURE 23 The social context of the doctor

I have spent my professional life working as a general practitioner in the English National Health Service (NHS). I am the product of a White, middle-class family with a Flemish Roman Catholic mother and an English Anglican father. My father was a trustee of a friendly society called The Ancient Order of Foresters. It was one of the forerunners of the welfare state, providing health and social insurance to working people who paid into a common fund against the vicissitudes of life and death. I was taught in a monastery school and studied medicine in London at Barts. I moved to Cambridge in 1978 and have lived there ever since. This is my social context. Liberal in outlook and socialist in political leaning, I have supported the ideal of the NHS throughout. Religion has come and gone in my life and now I believe in stardust: that's where I came from and that's where I'm headed. The state paid for my education and has paid my wages all my life and in return I have looked after the endless stream of people who have passed through my consulting room.

Every one of those patients has been seen through the prism of my life story. I have attempted to understand what each one has wanted and needed and to match my wit and resources to his or her predicament. The degree to which I have succeeded or failed has depended on my insight and knowledge, my capacity to suspend judgement and listen. My ability to help my patient has also crucially depended on the allocation of resources by the state through the NHS to my corner of the enterprise. The patient's ability to pay has never been a central factor in my work.

The NHS has been my professional social context. The most socially disadvantaged person on my list has had the same access to primary healthcare as the wealthy, educated adept who make up a large part of the population of Cambridge. I have been privileged to be exempted from the need to charge my patients directly or to treat them differently according to their means.

This extraordinary social construct – healthcare free at the point of use and funded from central government and financed by taxation – has become part of the fabric of our nation. It is part of our national story. Paying for a visit to the general practitioner is a fading folk memory. Society has moved a long way from the deference and gratitude of the post-war years and has adapted to business and profit, which now drives a desire for 24-hour access and the expectation of instant response. Capital and targets have replaced social responsibility and compassion. The social context of the consultation and the doctor has shifted too. Where previously there was a quiet space in which the patient could unfold his or her worries and symptoms there is now a crowd of imperatives. Doctors in all branches of medicine now face checklists, targets, time limits and output incentives, serviced by computer records with their prompts and demands. The currency of medicine has shifted away from the consultation as its gold standard, and process goals as surrogates for outcomes now have authority over many clinical decisions.

This is a fundamentally dehumanising change. When a target is the key indicator of performance, the individuality of the patient is in danger of being lost. The patient becomes an object to be manipulated, herded, sampled, tested or processed instead of a person to be respected, listened to and valued in his or her uniqueness of being and narrative.

The march of technology has meant that the cost of doing everything for everybody has far outstripped our ability to raise enough cash from taxation to pay for it. Rationing is far too adult a word to be mentioned by most politicians who can work only in brief electoral cycles, promising everything to an infantilised population who are never trusted to hear the truth and share their rightful place in facing up to the pain of saying no.

Box 50

Inevitable underfunding combined with denial of the need to ration makes a toxic cocktail when combined with a target-driven health economy obsessed with counting processes. The benighted practitioners at the front line (such as doctors and nurses in primary care and accident and emergency departments, healthcare assistants in nursing homes and on wards for the elderly, and many others across the NHS) are doomed to fail. Stressed, exhausted and demoralised, they cope by turning off their compassion, by denying the personhood of their patients and by becoming cynical and even callous. Scandalous failures of care are the bitter consequence.

These scandals are held up by politicians who blame the practitioners. Trust in the NHS is undermined and those with the means to do so, turn to private care. Providers deemed to have 'failed' are stripped of their contracts which are then sold to private bidders. These private providers have distant shareholders who care only about their dividends. Cheaper labour is imported and exploited. Standards fall further and care becomes fragmented. Ultimately, failing private providers leave gaping holes in the fabric of the NHS and the state is left to pick up the pieces, further straining what is left of the original concept of national care.

I am a passionate believer in the consultation as an antidote to all this gloom and chaos. The Synoptic View is a model that reminds the clinician that the predicament being presented must be seen as part of a complex system. The output of the consultation must be educated, wise, compassionate management. The patient must be guided towards the maximum possible autonomy, taking responsibility for his or her decisions and actions. The doctor must help the patient to become aware of as much reality as can be borne in relation to the problem under consideration. This will inevitably include cost constraint and societal attitudes.

Healthcare is very deeply political, because it flows from the decisions that citizens and their politicians make about priorities. The social context of doctors places a duty upon them to educate their patients and encourage them to take their share of responsibility for their health and the health of the society in which they live. The Synoptic View makes this duty clear and provides a framework for the adult discussion that perhaps we would all rather avoid.

CHAPTER 23

Dysfunction: The Social Context of the Illness

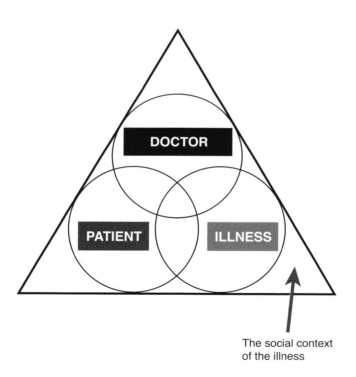

FIGURE 24 The social context of the illness

Disease categories and their names are a construct of society seeking to gain control over the inevitability of illness and eventual demise. Our quest for mastery over infections and infestations, cancers and senescence is accompanied by the vagaries of fashion and by the pursuit of gain.

Obesity, smoking and depression are phenomena that can illuminate the social contexts of illness.

In prehistoric times, food was hard to come by. Early humans had to scavenge for it, chase it and toil for it. As we have become more adept at manipulating our environment to suit ourselves, we have created leisure and abundance for ourselves. Two-thirds of the world's population is now sedentary and surrounded by food, while the other third is starving. Energy sources are stacked higher than our heads in our shops. Foods that are stuffed with sweetness and fats are very attractive to us because we are primed by our scavenging genes to gorge on these when we happen upon them. This was not a problem when such opportunities were rare and the energy bonus from finding wild honey or spearing a boar was a cause for celebration and communal feasting. Now we find sweetness and fats together in every bar of confectionery and we have become addicted to them. Our addiction is fuelled and encouraged by the food industry, which makes colossal profits from adding sugars and fats to our shopping baskets. We are victims of our tastes and we are passive in the face of exploitation by industry whose only purpose is domination through profit. Obesity and all its attendant woes are the predictable consequence. The prevalence of type 2 diabetes is soaring and doctors are rewarded for managing it in special clinics and with payments for meeting tick-box targets for eye checks and the like. In my surgeries I have felt like a minnow in a sea of self-inflicted illness as I have struggled to deal with morbidly obese people who are in despair at their condition and helplessness.

Proof of the harmfulness of smoking emerged from Richard Doll's work in the 1950s, based on research among doctors themselves.[73] The addictiveness of nicotine and the strenuous efforts of the tobacco industry have ensured that smoking remains popular and that young people are still recruited in every generation to line the pockets of the unscrupulous businesses that peddle heart attacks and cancer in glossy packages. The cohorts of the dead and diseased are replaced continually by the fresh-faced and the healthy, willing fodder for persuasion by advertising and peer pressure. Once again, doctors are faced with the consequences in their clinics and offices, swimming against a tide of self-harm that remains socially acceptable despite all the evidence of dreadful consequences. Even now, any move towards further control, such as plain packaging for cigarettes, is strenuously resisted by the entrenched tobacco industry, which seeks to manipulate politicians through shady lobbying and hidden patronage.

Psychopharmacology has existed for as long as the medicinal properties of plants have been recognised. Elders, shamans and apothecaries, quacks and physicians have all sought to harness mind-altering substances to further their quest for the relief of suffering for their supplicants. Every society and people has looked for ways to 'get out of their heads'. Cursed as we are with self-awareness and the foreknowledge of our own mortality, with memory and imagination, we suffer in a life that Thomas Hobbes described as 'solitary, poore, nasty, brutish, and short.'[74] Small wonder, then, that our patients are as keen to get their hands on such medicines as physicians are to prescribe them. In the middle part of the last century, drug treatment of mood disorder became possible with the advent of amphetamines, barbiturates and tranquillisers. People presenting to their doctors with the woes consequent upon lives that were indeed solitary, poor, nasty, brutish and short began to be offered relief in prescribed medication. To legitimise these prescriptions, anxiety neuroses, insomnia and mood disorders were diagnosed and new disorders were invented to match the expanding formulary of medications available. Drug companies were swift to assure prescribers that their products were harmless, non-addictive and effective. Evidence to the contrary was suppressed or ignored and biased studies entered the journals, conveniently omitting to mention adverse reactions or deaths related to these treatments. When, eventually, addiction reports and suicides mounted to levels that could no longer be hidden, the pharmaceutical industry sought less-dangerous compounds. Serotonin, the American name for the neurotransmitter known elsewhere as 5-hydroxytriptamine, entered the public consciousness and was deemed to be too low in many who consulted their physicians troubled by their life experiences. The scientific-sounding selective serotonin reuptake inhibitors were safer to prescribe and doctors were spared the trauma of their patients killing themselves with the very drugs that they had promised would make them happier. Advertising of these medications directly to the public reinforced the amine theory of depression and a new and exceptionally lucrative boom in prescribing followed.

Box 51

These three examples of the social context of illness have a common thread. The link is human suffering and our attempts to feel better. Alienation and loneliness, misery and feelings of inadequacy abound. We respond by seeking respite from these feelings in food, tobacco and antidepressants or tranquillisers. We ignore the long-term harm of these actions in order to escape momentarily from our predicament.

The Synoptic View of the consultation gives the doctor and the patient a chance of doing something different. The patient is met in his or her moment of need by a physician who is listening actively and who can synthesise the narratives as they unfold. The patient's story is given undivided attention and respect and the capacity of the patient for self-knowledge and healing is revealed. The illness is opened up to the knowledge, skill and values of both the doctor and the patient working together and the social contexts of the consultation are made explicit. At last, the patient has the experience of being held in mind, considered and valued – treated as unique in his or her quest for meaning and appropriate response to life's challenges. Pharmacology is put in its correct and limited place, the autonomy of the patient is enhanced and the loneliness and alienation at last acknowledged and addressed.

CHAPTER 24

Dysfunction: The Social Context of the Patient

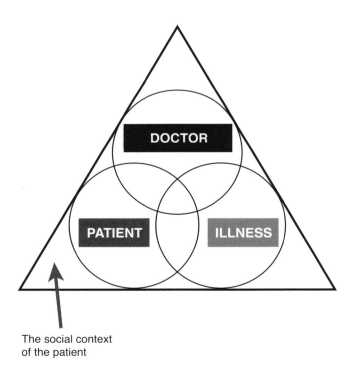

The social context
of the patient

FIGURE 25 The social context of the patient

In order to make sense of the world around us, we make observations and then make guesses and predictions based on our thoughts and judgements. Every person is his or her own anthropologist. Anthropologists look at societal behaviours and try to work out what rules are operating in the community under inspection and, mostly unconsciously, we do the same. If at first this sounds unlikely, think of the way children learn to talk. They listen intently for a year or so, and then hesitantly try out some nouns – 'mama, dada, dog', for example – and an occasional adjective such as 'hot' or adverb such as 'faster'. The child then goes on to construct short sentences that instinctively follow the grammatical rules of the language they are learning. They learn tenses and plurals, conditionals and qualifiers as if they were in an A-level foreign-language class, with no apparent effort. Within a year or two, they are fluent native speakers.

The consultation offers many opportunities for assumptions to be made about the social context of our patients. Traditional general practice is based on a registered list and typically the majority of patients live within a very short distance from the practice. The general practitioner gets to know the geographical area very quickly, and the connotations of each street name. As the doctor gains in local knowledge and experience, he or she will accumulate a store of stories about the patients in each area and will be making generalisations (or 'rules') by which to lay down a series of expectations. Just as insurance companies adjust their premiums by postcode, so doctors adjust their ideas and expectations by categorising their patients according to the social context implied by their address, speech patterns and clothes, body posture, age and every other clue that cascades from people and which is registered subconsciously and intuitively.

These pieces of information and the guesses that flow from them contribute to the doctor's story of the illness but they belong to the social context of the patient.

If the doctor makes wrong assumptions about the patient's social context or neglects to elicit sufficient information in this domain, consultations that otherwise would have produced excellent outcomes can go seriously awry.

Patients used to healthcare systems in which they pay the doctor directly for care often have very different expectations from patients who have been born and brought up in the National Health Service environment of care that is free at the point of use. In the National Health Service, the doctors by and large have no personal financial interest in their decisions about the investigations and treatments they recommend. In consequence, when faced with a self-limiting illness, deciding to do nothing, not to refer, not to investigate and not to treat is normal and this is accepted on trust. 'The doctor said I didn't need an X-ray . . . an antibiotic . . . a referral . . . .' In contrast, this judgement is often interpreted by patients trained in fee-for-service systems as uncaring, rejecting, dismissive and even negligent.

Box 52

A young mother once brought me a feverish infant having been up all night trying to pacify the miserable child who would not sleep. She told me her husband was angry at having his sleep disturbed, as he had to work all day. He had insisted she should come to the doctor. All seemed to go well as I listened to the mother's story of the illness and then carefully examined the child, following all the National Institute for Health and Care Excellence guidelines for the assessment of febrile children. The infant responded well to me and at the end of the examination all was smiles and confidence in the consulting room. When I outlined my management plan and explained that no prescription was needed and that the illness was likely to be self-limiting, the mother listened quietly. Then she got up and opened the door. She turned to me and delivered a tirade of criticism. She said that I was a heartless and unprofessional doctor – that I did not care about her infant's suffering or her husband's predicament. She lamented that she would not be able to face him when she returned empty-handed. She said that a doctor had never treated her so rudely and that she would never, ever see me again for anything. She demanded an immediate second opinion from a doctor who would 'at least prescribe a light antibiotic' and left to continue her complaint in the practice manager's office.

I had completely misjudged the social context of this consultation. The family were new arrivals in the UK from a fee-for-service system in which every illness any of them had ever had was treated with some form of medication. The idea that a sick child could leave a consultation empty-handed was utterly alien to them.

Until the moment the mother had launched her torrent of complaint, I had been congratulating myself upon a smoothly running surgery, and an exemplary consultation meeting all the requirements of our local microbiology department and guidelines from every authority ever to seek dominion over GP's management of minor illness.

This was a powerful lesson about the importance of the social context of consultation.

We may imagine we understand our patients, and my smug complacency was rewarded with a stinging rebuke, as I learned swiftly that my internal world is not to be projected upon my patients.

My duty as a doctor is to elicit the information necessary to meet the needs of the patient and the predicament with which they attend. Had I enquired more successfully about the ideas, concerns and expectations of this young mother and her husband, I might not have fallen into the trap that I set for myself. I would have sought to mould and educate, teach and encourage, reassure and offer resource, and gained an ally. Or I might still have got an earful for not prescribing the requisite antibiotic. Or perhaps I would have prescribed the antibiotic! At least I would have understood something vital for this consultation.

The Synoptic View has 10 domains. The social context of the patient is one of the most neglected areas of consultation and ignorance of these details is a frequent source of dissatisfaction, conflict and complaint. We may think we know what is in our patients' minds, or what their lives are like, or what their beliefs are, but we will sometimes get a very sharp reminder indeed that we are wrong – very wrong indeed. Each domain needs to be serviced by the consultation so that the information pertinent to the problem under consideration is elicited.

Part Three

Personal Reflections on Other Models of the Consultation

CHAPTER 25

Models of the Consultation

If I have seen a little further it is by standing on the shoulders of giants.

Sir Isaac Newton[75]

If I have not seen as far as others, it is because giants were standing on my shoulders.

Jeff Goll[76]

Our understanding of the GP consultation has evolved as the result of several important studies. In this final chapter I have briefly summarised some of the past models and ideas that have most influenced me. Reading them is like reading travel books before going to a foreign country – they are guides that can enrich our experience of exploring the Lonely Consultation.

1880: THE HOSPITAL MODEL

Until recently, nearly all medical teaching was undertaken in hospitals. The division of medicine into specialities emphasises the focus on organ-based disease. As I mentioned in Chapter 20, the caricature of the 'Liver in Bed 10' still has validity. Increasingly, however, the teaching of communication now gets priority in medical education. A substantial part of medical training is now undertaken in primary care.

The hospital model evolved from the application of the scientific method to disease. The model developed in the new teaching hospitals in Paris after the French Revolution. Patterns of disease were beginning to be better understood. The work of Giovanni Morgagni (1682–1771), the father of anatomical pathology, the invention of the stethoscope by René Laennec (1781–1826) and the insights of Ignaz Semmelweis (1818–65), Louis Pasteur (1822–95) and Robert

Koch (1843–1910) into the nature of contagion are just a few examples of the rapid expansion of scientific understanding of disease.

Box 53

The Hospital Model
- Disease
- Diagnosis
  - history
  - examination
  - tests
- Treatment

This new knowledge was hard-won. For many years doctors saw no reason to modify this approach. The hospital model has great strength, which is why it has survived intact into the age of molecular medicine. If you need a technical solution to a problem, the hospital model is well placed to provide it. Patients with cardiac chest pain can now get rapid relief after diagnosis and treatment with percutaneous insertion of a coronary artery stent.

The main drawback of the hospital model is that it tends to treat the patient as a specimen to be examined, just as the naturalists of the eighteenth and nineteenth century collected and catalogued the flora and fauna of the world.

The misapplication of the hospital model can lead to trouble. The individuality of the patient and the narrative of his or her illness, its meaning and social and emotional context can all get discounted. Tests can have false positives, treatments can be given inappropriately and side effects can complicate the situation.

Box 54

Adverse Effects of the Hospital Model

An anxious man of 30 with a long history of abdominal pains was admitted yet again to a teaching hospital as part of his unending search for a diagnosis. After 2 months of inpatient investigation the only abnormality found was delayed gastric emptying. He felt alienated by the staff because he was judged a 'difficult patient' and he found being in hospital demoralising and frightening. His exasperated medical team eventually discharged him home on more than 20 medications, including morphine. He was drowsy and depressed, and his abdominal symptoms were unabated. The hospital model had failed him and caused him to deteriorate.

1957: THE DOCTOR AS DRUG

He who asks questions will get answers, but hardly anything else.

Michael Balint[77]

When I arrived at my training practice in 1980 my trainers, Dr Piers Recordon and Dr Nigel Oswald, had fully absorbed the pioneering ideas of Michael Balint. Balint was a Hungarian psychoanalyst (and the son of a Budapest doctor) and worked, with his wife Enid, at the Tavistock Institute of Human Relations in London, where they ran discussion groups for GPs during the 1950s. Balint applied psychotherapeutic insights to the commonplace workings of general practice. For the first time, the interplay of feelings between the doctor and the patient were recognised to be important.

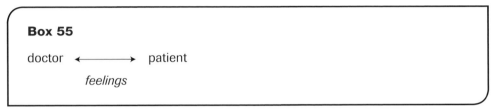

Box 55

doctor ←——→ patient
feelings

Balint recognised that the doctor himself was as much a treatment as any drug, and the idea of 'doctor as drug' emerged. He suggested that the specific role of the GP lay in understanding the whole of the patient's communication, and that the doctor's own feelings could be a key to unlock the meaning of the communication. The group became an attempt at 'enabling doctors to recognize and understand their patients' complaints, not only in terms of illnesses, but also in terms of personal conflicts and problems, and then to use this understanding so that it should have therapeutic effect'.[78]

Balint's ideas were initially very challenging to the profession. Some doctors were terrified by the idea that their own emotions might be exposed not only to others but also, most frighteningly of all, to themselves. Balint's teaching is now taken for granted as self-evident common sense. It is difficult to remember that these ideas were once so revolutionary and challenging.

Box 56

Balint Groups

Balint groups are alive and well today. In a Balint group a small group of GPs meets weekly to discuss difficulties with patients. They do so without notes and their description inevitably conveys some of their own subjective feelings. The group examines the doctor–patient interactions by asking the doctor questions. The doctor tends to take the role of his own patient, while the group assumes the role of the doctor. An underlying belief is that doctors are better able to listen to their patients if they have had the experience of being listened to sensitively themselves.

1964: TRANSACTIONAL ANALYSIS

We learn about being looked after from our parents. As children, we bring our aches and pains, our worries and our illnesses to our parents for reassurance and advice and treatment. It is not at all surprising then, that similar patterns appear when doctors and patients are working together as adults. It is very easy for doctors to become parental and patients to become childlike, instead of working together as adults.

Box 57

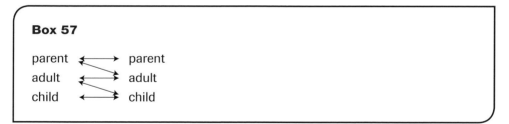

When we communicate, there is a flow of information at both conscious and unconscious levels. The exchange can be called a transaction. Eric Berne, a Canadian-born psychiatrist, recognised that transactions can be analysed to reveal the roles that people are playing when they are communicating. His influential book *Games People Play*[79] popularised his ideas. He suggested that we are all capable of behaving as Adults, Parents or Children in our dealings with one another, and that we play 'games' that have well-defined scripts.

I have found Berne's ideas especially helpful. His insights are constantly useful in my struggle to avoid falling into the traps of guilt, perfectionism and an exaggerated sense of responsibility that bedevil the work of the general practitioner.

We do best when we work as Adult to Adult, each taking responsibility for his or her thoughts, feelings and behaviour. Illness and disease can subvert our adult interactions and patients can present in a regressed, childlike state. This can be appealing and seductive to the doctor, who may respond in a parental fashion with authoritarian prescriptions and false reassurances. This risks impairment of the autonomy of the patient, and moves the locus of health control inappropriately towards the doctor. The patient avoids responsibility for the disease and becomes more dependent upon the doctor. These behaviours are self-reinforcing and infantilise the patient and trap the doctor in an exhausting and burdensome contract to make things better. Such an unrealistic contract is doomed to eventual failure, leading to guilt and recrimination and burnout.

For some patients, especially those who have suffered a deficit of good and loving parenting, attention from a doctor who exhibits parental behaviour can be very attractive and even addictive, locking them into a childlike state of dependency. Beware, then, of patients who bring you little presents, as a child might do, to please a parent. Like a cat that rubs itself around your legs at feeding time, there may be an ulterior motive!

Box 58

Examples of Parent, Adult and Child Interactions
Doctor: Have you been able to remember to take your medication?
Patient: Yes, I use a pill box with compartments to help me. **(Adult to Adult)**

Doctor: You really must remember to take your tablets!
Patient: I hate taking tablets! **(Parent to Child)**

Patient: You told me everything would be all right but now I have had a heart attack!
Doctor: If you had taken the medication properly this wouldn't have happened. **(Child to Parent)**

1972: 'PHYSICAL, PSYCHOLOGICAL, SOCIAL'

Those who are enamoured of practice without science are like the pilot who gets into a ship without rudder or compass and never has any certainty where he is going.

Leonardo da Vinci (1452–1519)[80]

In 1972 a working party from the Royal College of General Practitioners produced a report that helped to define general practice as a specialty. There were famous names among them, including Marshall Marinker, John Horder and

Donald Irvine. They recognised that future general practitioners had educational needs that were not being met by existing methods. Their report, *The Future General Practitioner: Learning and Teaching,*[81] contributed to the establishment of vocational training for general practitioners.

1972 was my first year at St Bartholomew's Hospital Medical School. I was already confident in my ambition to become a general practitioner, but the question my relatives often asked was: 'What do you want to specialise in?' 'Just a GP?' was their disappointed response to my assertion that this was the career I wanted.

Other disciplines within medicine had strong traditions of higher professional training and were able to assert their core of specialist knowledge. General practice had yet to achieve this goal. The *Future General Practitioner* set out a curriculum that for the first time described the content of general practice. In six chapters the authors set out their recipe for the education of the next generation of GPs. They described the underlying educational aims, the nature of the consultation and the way general practitioners used it to elicit, understand and meet patients' needs. They emphasised that the general practitioner had to understand the nature of health and disease, human development and behaviour, the role of medicine in society and the workings of practices and partnership itself.

The authors also described a problem-solving approach that remains helpful. They used the terms 'problems' and 'solutions' rather than the words 'diagnosis' and 'treatment', a new concept, and even suggested that doctors might examine a solution before implementing it – still a very useful piece of advice!

Box 59

A Problem-Solving Model
- Problem presented
- Problem examined
- Problem defined

- Solution proposed
- Solution examined
- Solution implemented

Their chapter on the consultation begins with a quotation from James Spence's (1892–1954) *The Purpose and Practice of Medicine,*[82] published in 1960:

The essential unit of medical practice is the occasion when, in the intimacy of the consulting room or sick room, a person who is ill, or believes himself to be ill, seeks the advice of a doctor whom he trusts. This is a consultation and all else in the practice of medicine derives from it. The purpose of the consultation is that the doctor, having gathered his evidence, shall give explanation and advice.

And the authors themselves commented:

it is our experience that an analysis of the consultation in these terms can often make clear to the trainee the process of a given consultation which he had previously found difficult to understand.[83]

They urged a problem-solving approach that involves making a hypothesis and taking action on it to test it. 'Imaginative conjecture and criticism, in that order, underlies the physician's diagnosis.'[84] Just in time for me, general practice had found its voice and a new specialty was becoming recognised.

1973: SIX MINUTES FOR THE PATIENT

Since the publication of his book *The Doctor, His Patient and the Illness*,[85] Michael Balint and his wife Enid had been extending their understanding of the general practice consultation using psychotherapeutic techniques. They recognised that it is easy for practitioners to become preoccupied with their own concerns in the consultation, leaving the patient's issues unexamined in the average 6-minute consultation.

Michael Balint died in 1970. In 1973 Enid and the group published *Six Minutes for the Patient*[86] based on case reports from GPs between 1966 and 1971 and which described techniques for getting closer to the real reason for the patient's problems. The group had examined and developed ways of offering psychological help to patients without disrupting the normal routine of practice. They described a phenomenon that they called the 'flash'.

Box 60

The Flash Technique
- Do not be too preoccupied with theories or preconceived questions (because you will miss the obvious in what the patient is saying)
- Observe intently and consider, and then make contact with what is bothering the patient at that moment
- Respect the patient's privacy but offer the opportunity for communication (and avoid the temptation force disclosures)

> The question is not whether a patient tries to communicate, but how much the doctor can respond to the communication. This is the difference between the detective technique and the flash technique, that the detective only collects material and understands it. How he responds to it is different, whereas the flash technique, if I'm right, is not only sensing what has happened and understanding, but responding, so doctor and patient should feel that their talk is the same language and not at cross purposes.
>
> Michael Balint[87]

Reading this work in 1979, I realised how little I understood of what was happening during consultations. I glimpsed something of the gap between the superficial label of the traditional diagnosis and a true therapeutic understanding of the patient's predicament. Fortunately, at the same time as I appreciated my own inadequacy in the task, these authors presented me with a simple technique that an ordinary general practitioner could use in everyday practice that would take me a little closer to my patient's real needs.

The Flash technique builds on continuity of care that general practice offers. Although individual consultations may be short, the Flash allowed insights that could be built upon in subsequent appointments, perhaps over many years. In Enid Balint's phrase: 'although the flash itself is brief the relationship in which it occurs is long.'

> Our experience shows that if these working principles are . . . adhered to an intense, intimate contact is sometimes made between the doctor and the patient. This contact does not lead to a dependent clinging relationship . . . but the flash of understanding, . . . may expose the tip of an iceberg or the heat of a fiery cauldron which perhaps . . . .. can gradually be explored. The therapy, we think, lies in the peculiar intense flash of understanding between the doctor and the patient in a setting where an ongoing contact is possible where neither the doctor nor the patient gives up his self esteem.
>
> Enid Balint[88]

Box 61

It is More Important to Make Contact . . .

A colleague was working in palliative care with a deeply withdrawn man with advanced and distressing facial cancer, who came to the hospice outpatient clinic every few weeks, never volunteering any information, always communicating with a passive and silent aggression. Finally the doctor felt driven to saying to him, 'Listening to you, I feel helpless and hopeless' and to his amazement the patient grinned, and from that moment real communication between them was much improved. By honestly sharing his feelings he had finally demonstrated empathy – by expressing the same feelings that he had himself – and it is empathy that is so often therapeutic.

1974: HEALTH BELIEF MODEL

There is nothing good or bad, but thinking makes it so.

William Shakespeare, *Hamlet* (act 2, scene 2)[89]

Why is it that people can come to such different conclusions when we all have access to more or less the same information? What accounts for the differences in the way people behave in the face of adversity and illness? In the 1950s a study of why people sought X-ray examinations for tuberculosis led to a recognition that deeply held beliefs influenced potential health-seeking behaviours.[90] Over the next 2 decades, this insight came to be known as the health belief model. Marshall Becker wrote a summary of the model in 1974.[91] In 1975, together with Lois Maiman, he published a review of the literature on the subject.[92] They attempted to find predictors of compliance within social and psychological variables. Their work identified some key areas of belief that would influence patients' behaviour.

Box 62

Health Belief Model
- Health interest
- Perceived vulnerability
- Perceived seriousness of the threat to health
- Costs and benefits of option
- Cues to action

When I have been baffled by the blind pig-headedness of the stubborn patient in front of me who steadfastly refuses to immunise her children, or give up smoking as his foot turns black, or seek help for the fungating breast cancer, I have turned to Becker and Maiman's work. It is only by going back to a patient's deeply (and sometimes unconsciously) held beliefs that such recalcitrance in the face of my obvious wisdom becomes intelligible.

Becker and Maiman noted that people vary considerably in their underlying interest in health issues: GPs know all about this. Some of our patients seem obsessed with their health, while others are blithe in the face of dire threat.

They observed that some people believe that they are invulnerable to illness while others take the opposite view and anxiously think that they will fall victim to anything and everything. Furthermore, they noted that people vary with respect to their beliefs about the seriousness of various illnesses and the risks of not having treatment. They observed that people came to different conclusions as they weighed up the pros and cons of each course of action that was proposed to them, evaluating the nuisance and risk of various courses of action. They also observed that external cues such as family events or publicity on television or in the press could influence health behaviour very strongly.

These five areas of health belief are strongly linked to the perceptions that people develop about the degree of control that they have over their health. This is the notion of the locus of health control. In people who perceive themselves to be in charge of their own health the centre of control (or locus) is believed to be inside them. In contrast, there are those who believe that they have no control over what happens to them, they are fatalistic or even nihilistic about their health. A third group attributes power over their health to another, perhaps the surgeon into whose hands they are committing themselves, or to a supernatural being, a god or a daemon.

Taken as a whole, these ideas lie within the patient's ideas, concerns and expectations. A good part of the 10 minutes of our consultations with our patients is taken up with eliciting these beliefs. Understanding what our patients believe and how they come to hold such beliefs gives us a privileged insight into their world and promotes mutual respect and tolerance.

Such understanding is an essential prerequisite to offering alternative perspectives and assessments that may lead patients to pursue paths to better health that they had previously discounted or believed impossible.

1975: HERON – SIX CATEGORIES OF COUNSELLING INTERVENTION

John Heron is a researcher and teacher who has devoted his career to studying processes within social encounters. Working in the 1970s with experienced GPs training to become trainers, he developed a model that helped to categorise and understand the types of interventions that a doctor can make when working with a patient. He defined an intervention as being 'an identifiable piece of verbal or non verbal behaviour that is part of the practitioner's service to the client'.[93]

Box 63

Six Categories of Counselling Intervention
Authoritative interventions:
1. prescriptive – seeking to direct the behaviour of the client
2. informative – imparting knowledge, information, meaning to the client
3. confronting – raising the client's consciousness about some limiting attitude or behaviour of which they are relatively unaware.

Facilitative interventions:
1. cathartic – seeking to enable the client to discharge, to abreact painful emotion, primarily grief, fear and anger
2. catalytic – seeking to elicit self-discovery, self-directed living, learning and problem-solving in the client
3. supportive – seeking to affirm the worth and value of the client's person, qualities, attitudes or actions.

The first three interventions are authoritative and dominant or assertive, while the second three seek an improvement in the patient's autonomy, nudging him or her to take more responsibility.

Early in my medical career I had become aware that the doctors I had worked with had a certain style. Some tended to be authoritative and paternalistic while others were more reflective and facilitative. Through Heron's work I understood that these styles were assembled from recognisable components. Furthermore, the interventions that characterised the styles could be learned and practised and applied consciously and in a way that best served the needs of the patient at that moment. In other words, the interventions could become part of a toolkit that a skilled clinician could draw upon as appropriate, rather than a stereotypical straightjacket of habit.

Heron went on to study the malfunctions that can occur when interventions are misguided or even malevolent. Each of the six categories has a dark side to it. The unwary or inept practitioner can fall into traps with his patient, causing harm and distress. The doctor may, for instance, press unsolicited attention on his patient or become manipulative, seeking his own interests. In other circumstances the doctor may compulsively project his or her own unresolved problems on the patient.

The doctor has a great deal of power during the consultation. With the best of intentions, prescriptive intervention could result in benevolent takeover, informative interventions could overwhelm the patient and confrontation could become aggression or poisonous undermining. The three facilitative interventions are no less likely to become twisted, with cathartic interventions being delivered in a way in which hurt is re-enacted, or buried distress becomes overwhelming. Catalytic interventions may probe obsessively, reflecting the doctor's need for order rather than the patient's search for meaning. Even supportive interventions can be corrupted with the patient being insultingly patronised.

Looking further into dysfunction, the interventions can be frankly malevolent. In the hands of those who seek to hurt or manipulate, coercion, lies and psychological attack, provocation, seduction and sedition are the weapons of the torturer, despot or dictator. The helping professions have their share of damaged and dangerous practitioners, since they are, after all, peopled by ordinary human beings.

Heron's work opened the door for me to an understanding of the seriousness of the work that I was undertaking. Verbal intervention is no less powerful a force than the apothecary's physic or the surgeon's knife. He who wields it had better know what he is doing. We owe it to our patients to look out for our own unmet needs and to be vigilant for the signs of malpractice around us.

1976: BYRNE AND LONG – *DOCTORS TALKING TO PATIENTS*

> *We had the experience but missed the meaning,*
> *And approach to the meaning restores the experience*
> *In a different form, . . .*
>
> TS Eliot, Four Quartets[94]

When I arrived at my first training practice in 1980 I was introduced to a new way of thinking about patients. The partnership had a psychodynamic approach to consultation – always keen to see beneath the surface and consider what was actually meant by what was said and done. I was given Byrne and Long's astonishing book *Doctors Talking to Patients*[95] to read. Patrick Byrne was a founder member of the College of General Practitioners. He and Barry Long, a psychologist, had done something very simple – they audiotaped what was said in the consulting room and then transcribed it. What they discovered was shocking. For a good part of the time, the doctor and the patient were not communicating. It was not only that they were not listening to each other: at times each quite literally had no idea what the other was talking about.

If you have ever listened to *The Archers* on Radio 4 you may have noticed that characters from Ambridge constantly fail to notice the most obvious cues that major misunderstandings are in train. Furthermore, characters are entrenched in roles that often approach caricature. This enriches the plot by allowing it to become more convoluted and enhances the enjoyment of the listener who can experience the tension of evolving drama with the privilege of knowing what is really going on.

Doctors and patients who miss cues during consultation suffer the same fate as the inhabitants of Ambridge – doomed to become entangled in misunderstanding and cross purposes, baffled by incomprehension and prejudice.

Until Byrne and Long's book revealed the truth, doctors had believed themselves to be skilled communicators, eliciting histories and imparting wisdom reliably and in a disciplined way. Far from it! The gap in communication between doctor and patient was often very wide and remained unbridged and unperceived in many of the consultations Byrne and Long recorded. The recordings showed that most doctors exhibited rigid and stylised consultation styles and speech patterns – regardless of the needs of the patient in front of them.

Following their example, I audiotaped some of my own faltering consultations. Unsurprisingly, my recordings revealed the spectrum of miscommunications: failing to hear, talking across each other, incomplete sentences, symptoms and observations ignored, instructions inadequate and information lacking – to name but a few.

Byrne and Long suggested a structure for the consultation that would help the doctor and the patient to understand each other better – at least the framework might help a lost doctor to find his or her way from the beginning to the end of the consultation. Unsurprisingly, they noted that failure to manage the second task – attempting to discover the reason for the patient attending – was associated with more frequent miscommunication.

Trainees in medicine are now used to video recordings, audio recordings, actors simulating consultations, role play and a variety of ways of observing and replaying the interaction between the doctor and the patient with a view to enhancing their communication skills. In 1976, this was revolutionary.

Box 64

Six Tasks Within the Consultation
1. Establish the relationship
2. Attempt to discover the reason for attending
3. Examination – verbal and/or physical
4. Reflect on the condition
5. Advise on treatment or tests
6. Terminate the interview

1979: STOTT AND DAVIS – THE EXCEPTIONAL POTENTIAL . . .

Doctors in working in general practice were coming to appreciate both the complexity and the potential of those few minutes spent between the doctor and the patient. General practice was emerging as a fully fledged specialty. Perhaps there was a hope that my aunts would stop asking me why I was 'just a GP . . .'

Writing in the *Journal of the Royal College of General Practitioners*, Stott and Davis from the Welsh National School of Medicine described 'The exceptional potential of each primary care consultation'.[96] They suggested that every contact between the doctor and his patient offered opportunities for work in four distinct areas and proposed the diagram shown in Box 64 as an aide-memoire.

Box 65

Area A Identification and management of the presenting problem	Area B Management of continuing problems
Area C Modification of the patient's help seeking behaviour	Area D Opportunistic health promotion

---

The job was clearly more complex than my aunts realised. Perhaps they should have been suggesting I do something easy like becoming a specialist rather than grappling with the impossible imperatives of primary care.

Stott and Davis were concerned to help both trainees and established practitioners by developing a

> concept of the practical potential in every single consultation in primary care which can be easily memorised, understood and used.

While I was a trainee attending the weekly day-release course in Cambridge, this framework was adopted as a lens through which our consultations could be examined. Stott and Davis had hoped that their aid would become a useful theoretical base, highlighting unique features of general practice, a teaching tool and a framework for discussion of the philosophy and principles of primary care. This hope became a reality for us. They had seen that

It is too easy to treat each presenting problem but fail to perceive the manipulations or cries for help which lie behind successive acute episodes of minor illness.

They showed that what is all too easily dismissed as mundane, trivial or even boring minor illness could be redefined as rich, patterned and meaningful.

All of this resonated strongly with my own ambitions for a career in general practice. They articulated my aspiration that each consultation should

ensure that the patient leaves better able to make informed choices.[97]

Stott and Davis's short paper reinforced my career choice and set me thinking along the paths that led to my own attempt at creating an aide-memoire for the consultation.

1981: HELMAN – FOLK BELIEFS

In 1981 Cecil Helman published a paper entitled 'Disease Versus Illness in General Practice',[98] which invited doctors to consider the experience of illness from the patient's perspective. Helman was born in Cape Town, from a long line of rabbis and doctors. He moved to the UK and became a general practitioner in London. He developed an interest in anthropology and went on to become professor of medical anthropology at Brunel University. Helman observed that disease and illness were models or 'ways of constructing reality, of imposing meaning on the chaos of the phenomenological world.'[99] Doctors and patients have different perspectives and needs when constructing their versions of reality. Each seeks to reduce the anxiety that accompany the chaos and complexity and arbitrary contingency of human experience. Helman quotes Cassell,[100] who says: 'I shall use the word "illness" to mean what the patient feels when he goes to the doctor's office, and "disease" to mean what the patient has after leaving the doctor. Disease, then, is something an organ has; illness is something a man has.'

Helman goes on to explore the idea of folk models of illness and suggests that all people have six questions whose answers will shape the illness and the behaviour of the patient and those around him or her.

Box 66

Helman: The Six Questions of Folk Models of Illness
1. What has happened?
2. Why has it happened?
3. Why to me?
4. Why now?
5. What would happen if nothing were done about it?
6. What should I do about it – or whom should I consult for further help?

Faced with observations of dysfunction, the six questions will lead the person with illness to seek answers from within their own cultural circle and resources. As clinicians we are prone to imagine that we are as important and central in our patients' minds as we are in our own, but only when 'the patient and those around them feel unable to deal with the illness is it brought to the general practitioner, to be converted into disease.'[101]

When we meet our patients we struggle to understand what they are saying. We may think we understand their words, but do we understand their meaning and context? We can improve our ability to understand and engage with our patients' predicaments by knowing that they will be asking themselves the six questions and constructing a folk model of their illness with the answers. Helman published poetry too. In his poem 'Hieroglyphics',[102] Helman muses upon the difficulty of understanding what is said by someone from another culture.

Box 67

'Hieroglyphics' (A Prose Poem by Cecil Helman)

She speaks to me in hieroglyphics. In a row of tiny pictures. Each one brightly coloured. And finely detailed. Each picture never quite straight, always facing sideways. She speaks quickly, one image following another. A long row of them, and then more after that. Her hair is dark as Anubis, her blue eyes of Horus outlined in black. A golden cobra lies coiled around her head. Whenever she speaks, I find myself mesmerized by this endless row of images. Crafted in arcane language, one after the other. A row of brightly-painted hieroglyphics. I wish I knew what she was trying to say.

I was attracted by the narrative implied by Helman's exploration of folk models of illness. If I wished to be of help to my patients, I would need to be able to encourage storytelling and to get my patients to trust me sufficiently to tell me about the answers they had already worked out for themselves. I would need to understand their perception of the need that had led them to consult and I would have to construct answers to their questions that were intelligible in the terms they were using to create meaning for themselves in a baffling world.

Cecil Helman respected his patients' expertise. He was among the first to acknowledge that authority over an illness is different from authority over a disease. Such authority was not easily gained and impossible without the patient's perspective.

1984: PENDLETON – IDEAS, CONCERNS AND EXPECTATIONS

By now, with vocational training firmly at the heart of medical education for a career in primary care a new generation of family doctors was being taught to consider the patient's perspective. Building on Byrne and Long's work with audiotaped consultations, the advent of video recording had made it possible to see as well as hear what went on in the consulting room. Pendleton and his colleagues in Oxford took Stott and Davis's aide-memoire for the four areas of the consultation (presenting complaint, management of ongoing problems, modification of help-seeking behaviour and opportunistic health promotion) and produced a checklist of tasks for the consultation.[103]

Box 68

The Consultation: an Approach to Learning and Teaching
1. To define the reasons for the patient's attendance, including:
    i.   the nature and history of the problems
    ii. their aetiology
    iii. the patient's ideas concerns and expectations
    iv. the effects of the problems
2. To consider other problems
    i. continuing problems
    ii. at-risk factors
3. To choose with the patient an appropriate action for each problem
4. To achieve a shared understanding of the problems with the patient
5. To involve the patient in the management and encourage him to accept appropriate responsibility
6. To use time and resources appropriately
7. To establish or maintain a relationship with the patient that helps to achieve the other tasks.

Pendleton's seven tasks emphasised the need for the doctor to do more to ensure that the reason for the patient's attendance was elicited. Pendleton understood the folk model and the questions that the patient would have asked him- or herself. He recognised that the general practitioner would need to put extra effort into getting the patient to reveal the fruits of his or her thinking. Pendleton summarised this with the formula 'ideas, concerns and expectations', now so familiar that it is hard to imagine a time when this mantra was unknown!

I was already familiar with audio-taping my consultations and soon I was experimenting with video. I watched with embarrassment as my tics and quirks were played and replayed, with all my errors and omissions exposed to the scrutiny of my teachers and peers. It was clearer than ever as we studied the consultation that it contained; complexity that went way beyond the linear models we were studying. Far from being able to start at the beginning, work through a series of tasks and finish at the end with a neat summation and prescription, my consultations wove backwards and forwards between history and advice, examination and prescription as I tried to get a grip on what it was the Royal College was expecting me to achieve and what the patient needed.

Pendleton recognised that using video recordings in teaching exposed the doctor to risk of destructive criticism, embarrassment and ridicule. In order to make it safer for the doctor, Pendleton suggested a sequence of events for consultation analysis:

1. learner and teacher observe and usually map the consultation
2. the learner and teacher observe and briefly clarify any matters of fact
3. the consultation is evaluated using the rating scale
4. the learner discusses those tasks which, in his opinion, were achieved
5. the teacher or other observers discuss those tasks which, in their opinions, were achieved
6. the learner discusses those tasks which, in his opinion were not achieved
7. the teacher or other observers discuss those tasks which, in their opinions, were not achieved and make their recommendations
8. disagreements are discussed and, if possible, resolved.

The learner is left with a clear summary of his strengths and of those specific changes that might lead to improvement. As learners become more comfortable with their peer group and less embarrassed about seeing themselves on the screen, it is possible to shortcut by moving swiftly to focus on the key concerns of the doctor who has been recorded and of the patient as perceived by the observers.

The consultation that had once looked easy had now become almost impossibly complex. I was daunted by the size of the task to be completed in the few minutes allotted to each patient. My head was spinning with lists and exhortations, agendas and models. How could the job be done? And could it ever be done well? Perhaps aspiring to be a good general practitioner is a manifestation of a psychotic omnipotence fantasy.

1987: NEIGHBOUR – *THE INNER CONSULTATION*

By the early nineties I had been a partner for several years and was keen to train as a trainer. I had cut my teeth on a diet of Balint, Byrne and Long, Helman and Pendleton but now I was going to be the teacher. Luckily, an influential book entitled *The Inner Consultation*[104] by Watford GP Roger Neighbour had come to the fore.

Neighbour accurately described the predicament that I was experiencing: my head was stuffed with the theory of what I should be achieving and this was getting in the way of what I should be doing. As Neighbour put it, 'It's not that I don't know what to do, it's that I don't do what I know.' What was making it more difficult was that I had now taken on the responsibility of training a new general practitioner. How could I teach them to do what I could not do myself? Neighbour helpfully suggested that I might think of myself being in two minds – having two heads. One head would be the Organiser and the other would be the Responder. The first would look after the structure of the consultation and the second would manage the non-verbal, intuitive, associative and creative responses that good consultation needs. He went on to describe a 'simple way of moving smoothly through a consultation, via five "checkpoints."'

His memorable drawing of a hand with the digits labelled with the names of the five checkpoints is likely to be recognisable instantly by the majority of GPs working in Britain today. The checkpoints are:

1. Connect
2. Summarise
3. Handover
4. Safety Net
5. Housekeeping.

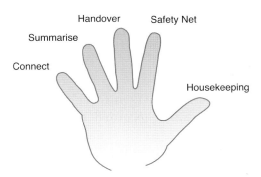

FIGURE 26 The five checkpoints

These checkpoints mapped to the consultation models that have already been considered but in a colloquial way that enabled me to have a quieter mind. This allowed me a more open space in which to engage with the patient, without worrying so much about a doctor-oriented, task-based agenda in which I was bound to fail and likely to alienate my patient. My two heads could work together cooperatively supported by a framework giving method and structure and boundary to the consultation. It was safe to practise again.

- **Connect.** The first phase of the consultation is about greeting a patient properly, putting him or her at ease and paying attention. It is also about determining the reason that the patient is there and hearing and understanding his or her story.
- **Summarise.** The next phase is about checking with the patient that you have understood him or her correctly, sorting things out in your own mind and making a plan.
- **Handover.** This is about giving the benefits of the consultation back to the patient. It may mean literally the handover of a prescription or it may mean the handover of knowledge. It is also about giving responsibility back to the patient as the patient leaves you to take up his or her life on his or her own again.
- **Safety Net.** This phase of the consultation deals with the 'What If?' questions. It is about looking with patients at possible outcomes, such as getting better or worse or needing an urgent contact and the need for follow-up.
- **Housekeeping.** This idea is partly about having a tidy desk with the notes adequately written but it is also about making sure that you are in a reasonable shape physically and emotionally for the next consultation. If you are drenched in sweat and palpitating with anxiety after a frightful confrontation with the last patient, it is not a good idea to go straight into the next consultation without taking a breather.

Neighbour divided his book into three sections: goal setting, skill building and 'getting it together'. He emphasised that the core skills of consulting could be defined, taught and practised and he articulated a holistic, integrated style of general practice that inspired a generation of doctors.

1989: COHEN-COLE AND BIRD – THE THREE-FUNCTION APPROACH TO THE MEDICAL INTERVIEW

As medical education broadened to include a wider understanding of the consultation, there was a need for a comprehensive textbook of the skills to be taught and learned. Leading the way were Steven Cohen-Cole, a physician from

Alabama, and Julian Bird, a UK physician and psychiatrist. They developed the *three-function* approach to the medical interview.[105]

While many consultation guides concentrate on gathering data to understand the patient's problems, Cohen-Cole and Bird included a new emphasis on the skills that are necessary in order to empathise with patients and to educate and motivate them. In the disease-focused models of old, it was presumed that the physician embodied the skills and attributes necessary for the practice of the art of medicine. Increasingly it was clear that these skills and attributes were not innate but could be described, taught and practised. The authors drew on examples from their own experience to provide the material to analyse and illustrate their ideas and they emphasised the teachability of the individual skills that they identified as necessary for successful consultation.

Their *three functions* can be summarised as:

1. gathering data to understand the patient's problems
2. developing rapport and responding to patient's emotion
3. patient education and motivation.

Cohen-Cole and Bird suggested that specific skills were needed for each of the three functions.

- **Gathering data**:
  - open-ended questions
  - narrowing the questions down as needed
  - facilitation
  - checking
  - overview of problems identified with negotiation of priorities
  - clarification and summarising
  - eliciting ideas and expectations
  - assessment of impact of diseases on quality of life.
- **Developing rapport**:
  - reflection
  - legitimation
  - support
  - partnership
  - respect.
- **Education and motivation**:
  - education about disease
  - agreeing a plan of action
  - motivation of the unwilling.

The three-function model has been taken up widely in the United States, and Cohen-Cole and Bird's book is standard fare for medical students there. Close emphasis on the structure and function, nature and quality of the consultation, previously the concern of general practitioners and psychiatrists, had become part of the core curriculum for all doctors.

1996: TEACHING COMMUNICATION SKILLS – THE CALGARY– CAMBRIDGE GUIDE

Despite Cohen-Cole and Bird's work, it was still not generally accepted that the central skills of successful communication could be taught. Fortunately, there were clinical teachers who had a more optimistic and practical approach. At Calgary in Canada and at Cambridge in the UK, medical training schemes had a tradition of giving central importance:

> to attending to both disease (the symptoms and signs, diagnostic reasoning, and biomedical understanding that characterise Western medicine) and illness (the unique experience of the individual patient – or his or her ideas, concerns, expectations, feelings, and thoughts) in every consultation.[106]

Professor Suzanne Kurtz from the faculty of medicine in Calgary and Dr Jonathan Silverman and Dr Juliet Draper, general practitioners from Cambridge, comprehensively showed that communication skills could be taught, in two linked volumes: *Teaching and Learning Communication Skills in Medicine*[107] and *Skills for Communicating with Patients*.[108]

These exhaustively researched books demolish all suggestions that consultation skills are innate and cannot be taught. Building on published literature and their own experience with their colleagues, Kurtz, Silverman and Draper have written the definitive guide for teachers of communications skills and those seeking to understand and improve communication with their patients.

In *Teaching and Learning Communication Skills in Medicine* the authors consider how a curriculum for communication skills might be constructed, and define the core content of such skills. They then anatomise the range of teaching and learning methods appropriate to students in this field. Throughout, there is a consistent appeal to the principles, concepts and research evidence for teaching communication skills and a steady focus on what is practical.

The book is divided into three sections: the first examines what is to be taught, the second considers how the principles may be applied in practice and the third looks at the social context of communication skills teaching.

In *Skills for Communicating with Patients*, Silverman, Kurtz and Draper define the overall curriculum of skills for consultation. They lay out the whole toolkit that a clinician might be called upon to use and show when and how the various tools might be used, their value and purpose, and the evidence for their effectiveness. They show how the practitioner can assemble the skills to benefit the patient and improve the outcome of the consultation.

Both books use the Calgary–Cambridge observation guide as a framework for thinking about the consultation, analysing its structure and understanding the role of each skill required to achieve the best outcome for the patient. The guide builds on the models presented by earlier authors.

Box 69

The Calgary–Cambridge Observation Guide to the Consultation
- Initiating the session
  - establishing initial rapport
  - identifying the reason(s) for the consultation
- Gathering information
  - exploration of problems
  - understanding the patient's perspective
  - providing structure to the consultation
- Building the relationship
  - developing rapport
  - involving the patient
- Explanation and planning
  - providing the correct amount and type of information
  - aiding accurate recall and understanding
  - achieving a shared understanding: incorporating the patient's perspective
  - planning: shared decision-making
  - options in explanation and planning
- Closing the session

Within the plan, each task is expanded into a framework for identifying the individual skills of the consultation. In all, 70 separate skills are identified.

The consultation is at the very heart of general practice, and communication skills are at the centre of that heart. These two inspiring and daunting books humble the reader (well, me anyway). Who among us dares to assert that we do this job well? With keen awareness of my deficits among the 70 skills, I am all too sensible of what is at stake when I start my surgery each day. I am constantly grateful for the kindness and forgiveness of my patients as I share with them the struggle to understand each other. Together, these volumes are a tour de force of analysis and clarity, and show what can be achieved when academic rigour is brought to bear on consultation skills learning and teaching. They both inspire me to do better and show me the way forward.

1998: GREENHALGH AND HURWITZ – *NARRATIVE BASED MEDICINE*

> The act of telling a story to the listener changes the story. Just as one cannot step into the same river twice, the narrator cannot ever tell exactly the 'same' narrative again . . .. On the listener's side, none of us ever truly 'hears' a story exactly as it is told by the narrator. Each story inevitably has gaps of meaning and significance, and we fill in these gaps as we imagine the world to be and as we imagine the teller intended. Thus, rather than hear a story, it is rather more accurate to say that we construct for ourselves a story about what we think we are hearing.
>
> Howard Brodie, foreword to *Narrative Based Medicine*[109]

This inspiring book resonated with the consulting style that I was evolving as I continued my work as a general practitioner. I relished the frank directness of storytelling that my patients brought me – a new one every 10 minutes or so. Work that might have seemed trivial, repetitive or mundane if stripped of the personal and rendered into the cold facts of the medical history was instead rich and varied, unique every time. *Narrative Based Medicine* celebrates this perception, starting with stories of illness that paint rich pictures of real people trying to make sense of what was happening to them – tumours, strokes, epilepsy.

The book is a compendium of many authors' thoughts about the narrative, and Sir Richard Bayliss takes the reader onwards from the patient's story to consider the behaviour of the medical listener:

> Not only must the physician hear what is said but with a trained ear he or she must *listen* to the exact words that the patient uses and the sequence in which they are uttered. In addition patients use another method of communication – body language – of which they are usually quite unconscious. The recipient of the narrative must keep both ears and eyes open to receive these two equally important complementary narratives.
>
> Sir Richard Bayliss[110]

Iona Heath[111] emphasises the unique role of the general practitioner as a listener to whom the patient can return again and again:

> For many patients, the general practice record, whatever its limitations, is the only sustained written record of their lives. The existence of this concrete documentation of their suffering, coping and endurance gives tangible form to the general practitioner's role as witness the patient's unfolding life story.

And she describes the role of the physician in helping the patient to make sense of what is happening:

Once the technical transactions of medicine are complete, general practitioner and patient still have to come to terms with the debility, pain and fear that comes with illness and disease.[112]

John Launer,[113] who went on to co-edit later editions of *Narrative Based Medicine*, introduces the idea that narrative-based medicine may sometimes be able to give patients the resources to retell their story in a new way to themselves, unlocking resources and freeing themselves from burdens carried for decades. He says:

> In my clinical GP work I am aware of narrative in three of its aspects:
> * in its familiar role in taking a traditional medical history
> * in its counselling aspect, as something which needs to be listened to, allowing patients to give coherence to their own history
> * as a therapeutic stance which involves questioning the patient in a way that *explores new meaning which may make a difference to the patient.*

Among other gems I found in this book, Glyn Elwyn and Richard Gwyn offer a glimpse of discourse analysis as a tool to examine the minutiae of the interaction between the patient and the doctor, reminding me of the fractal nature of the consultation when it is under the microscope, and Trisha Greenhalgh suggests that a narrative approach offers a way out of the frustration that primary care doctors experience when they try to apply evidence-based research findings to real-life case scenarios.

2007: MOULTON – *THE NAKED CONSULTATION*

During the long gestation of my own book about the consultation (at least six times longer than the gestation of the African Elephant), new books about the art of being a general practitioner have appeared from time to time. None is better than *The Naked Consultation*.[114] Liz Moulton is a contemporary of mine and her journey of discovery of the mysteries of the consultation appears to parallel my own. Her comprehensive and accessible guide to the literature, learning and practice of consultation skills is an ideal companion for any clinician. It wears its considerable authority lightly and is suitable for every stage of learning. Medical students, GP registrars, new principals and old-timers can all benefit from the engaging, unstuffy and practical wisdom within these pages.

The Naked Consultation approaches the interaction between clinician and patient from two perspectives. In the first part, Liz Moulton anatomises the consultation and reflects on the processes at work and the tools and skills needed to achieve a satisfactory outcome. In the second part, she tackles the teaching and learning of skills, the techniques used in training and the requirements of the Membership of the Royal College of General Practitioners (MRCGP) examination and subsequent appraisals.

2008: STUART AND LIEBERMANN – *THE FIFTEEN MINUTE HOUR*

A splendidly useful nugget that I collected from *The Fifteen Minute Hour*[115] was the BATHE model for dealing with patients who are experiencing intense emotion. One of the troublesome consequences of good consulting is that patients reveal their feelings to you! What do you do with the outpourings that may result?

Although this model might seem simplistic, it is based on very effective brief psychotherapeutic techniques. It actively discourages the patient from developing dependency on the doctor (bad for both patient and doctor) and instead helps the patient to explore realistic coping strategies. It is a model that works with and supports the patient's own coping strategies (however embryonic), and encourages further development of coping skills and responsibility for their own behaviours, feelings and actions.

Box 70

The BATHE model
- Background
- Affect
- Trouble
- Handling
- Empathy

Background
Question: **'What is going on in your life right now?** This question helps you to understand the patient's situation. The qualifying phrase 'right now' helps the patient to focus on the here and now.

Affect
Question: **'How do you feel about that?'** This moves the patient forward from a description of events. It acts as a punctuation mark in the patient's thoughts so that he or she can tell you more easily what is specifically causing him or her problems.

Trouble
Question: **'What is troubling you most?'** This is a focusing tool that will help the patient to tell you what it is that is really getting on top of him or her. The key word is 'most', and the patient's response to the question can lead you to the central problem.

Handling

Question: 'How are you handling this?' This question has two effects. First, it moves the problem forward again from defining it clearly into talking about actions. Second, it also has an implicit meaning (a presupposition) that the patient is handling it. In other words, it shifts responsibility for the problem back to the patient. This is useful for both apparently helpless patients and also for well meaning, but overhelpful, clinicians.

Empathy

Statement: 'I can understand that this must be difficult for you.' This empathic remark helps to balance the practical nature of the other parts of the model. Equally it expresses caring and concern without implying that the clinician can make it better or has a solution, or that the patient should hand over responsibility for the problem to the clinician.

2009: NAIDOO AND MONKLEY – *CONSULTATION SKILLS FOR THE NEW MRCGP*

There is nothing quite like the challenge of an examination for focusing the mind. An objective opinion from an impartial observer, armed with a marking schedule and authorised by a Royal College brings the 10-minute consultation down to the ground with a bump.

Can you do it?

Naidoo and Monkley's highly practical book *Consultation Skills for the New MRCGP*[116] is written for candidates for the MRCGP examination and comes with a DVD of 13 consultations. The book is divided into three sections. The authors present two assessment frameworks: the Clinical Skills Assessment and the Clinical Observation Tool, used by examiners to judge the performance of candidates.

The first section uses the DVD and invites the reader to judge the consultations using a Clinical Skills Assessment marking schedule and decide whether the doctor:
- 'asked the right questions, at the right time, in the right way
- performed the right examination correctly
- communicated in a precise, understandable and sensitive manner'.[117]

I found these consultations very convincing and real. They reminded me just how challenging the 10-minute consultation can be. You never know what is coming next, you always need more time, and you could always do with more expertise. I particularly liked the ninth consultation about pre-wedding diet pills and the thirteenth about allergy tests. Saying no in general practice is harder than saying yes, and to shift a patient's expectations requires particular skill and sensitivity if the patient is to remain fully engaged. Each consultation has a debrief by the authors with which to compare your own judgement and offers advice about relevant literature or internet resources underlying the points raised in the consultation.

The second section of the book gives twenty scenarios for use in role-play consultations, raw material for practice and assessment using the Clinical Skills Assessment and the Clinical Observation Tool. The cases are presented with crib sheets for the participants. The crib sheet for the person playing the doctor role sets out the brief for the clinician, gives some background information about the patient and lists the key tasks for the consultation. The crib sheet for the patient role gives the outline of the problem and some background and character information. It coaches the role-player in responses to likely scenarios that may emerge in the course of the consultation as the doctor tries to meet the patient's needs and to manage the consultation. Each case then concludes with notes about:

- data gathering, examination and clinical assessment skills
- clinical management skills
- interpersonal skills: know and treat this patient.

The cases cover a wide range of general practice competencies and working through them will provide excellent practice for both the MRCGP examination and real life. For those who enjoy a multiple-choice question, each case has a theoretical knowledge quiz. Suggestions for further reading are also included. The 20 cases can also be used for individual study by writing down the questions the clinician would need to ask of the patient, and then referring to the additional information for the patient's role as necessary.

In the third section of the book, the authors present mock cases for use in the Clinical Skills Assessment of the MRCGP examination. The format is similar to the second section, and presents a series of consultations that might be included in the mock surgery of 13 patients that examination candidates will have to undertake. Once again, there is a brief for the doctor and for the patient, a debrief, and a multiple-choice question followed by suggestions for additional reading. The task for the doctor in every case is to:

> **integrate** and **apply** clinical, professional, communication and practical skills appropriate for general practice, 'to produce a consultation that is meaningful to both patient and doctor and which moves the patient forward towards a justifiable management of their presenting problem'.[118]

If the ideas that I have presented here in *The New Doctor, Patient, Illness Model: Restoring the Authority of the GP Consultation* help you with your consultations in the future, assisting you in meeting the challenge of general practice, then I shall be richly rewarded knowing that I have contributed in some small way to the benefit that your patients undoubtedly derive from consulting you.

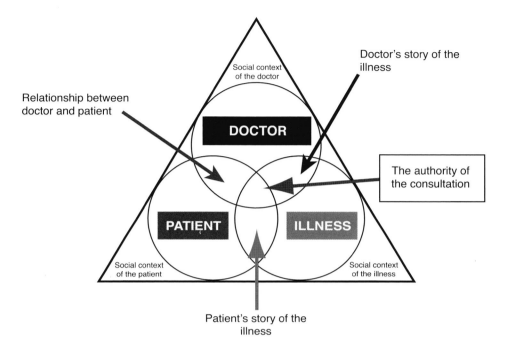

FIGURE 27 The Synoptic View of the consultation

References

1 Nadal D. *Lute Songs of John Dowland: the original first and second books/transcribed for voice and guitar*. New York: Dover Publications Inc; 1997.

2 *Oxford English Dictionary*. Oxford: Oxford University Press; 1971.

3 Working Party of the Royal College of General Practitioners. *The Future General Practitioner*. London: Royal College of General Practitioners; 1972.

4 Westcott R. Consultation models. *Doctor*. 2005; Sep 13: p. 43.

5 Shakespeare W. As you like it. Act 5, scene 1. In: *William Shakespeare The Complete Works*. Wells S, Taylor G, editors. Oxford: Oxford University Press; 1988. p. 648.

6 Balint M. *The Doctor, His Patient and the Illness*. 2nd ed. London: Churchill Livingstone; 2000.

7 Hippocrates. *The Book of Prognostics*. Hippocrates Vol II, Loeb Classical Library No. 148. Jones WHS, translator. Harvard, MA: Harvard University Press; 1923.

8 Stacey R. *Managing the Unknowable: strategic boundaries between order and chaos in organizations*. San Francisco, CA: Jossey-Bass; 1992.

9 Ibid.

10 Working Party of the Royal College of General Practitioners, op. cit.

11 Monod J. *Chance and Necessity: an essay on the natural philosophy of modern biology*. London: Vintage; 1971.

12 Ibid.

13 Peck MS. *The Road Less Travelled: the new psychology of love, traditional values and spiritual growth*. London: Rider; 1988.

14 World Health Organization (WHO). *Constitution of the World Health Organization*. New York, NY: WHO; 1946.

15 Ibid.

16 McWhinney I. The need for a transformed clinical method. In: Stewart M and Roter D, editors. *Communicating with Medical Patients*. Newbury Park, CA: Sage Publications. 1989.

17 The order for the burial of the dead. In: *The Book of Common Prayer*. Oxford: Oxford University Press; 1969. p. 395.

18 Blake W. Auguries of innocence. In: Ostriker A, editor. *The Complete Poems*. London: Penguin Classics; 1977. p. 506.

19 Mandelbrot B. How long is the coast of Britain? Statistical self-similarity and fractional dimension. *Science*. 1967; **156**(6): 636–8.

20 Carroll L. Tweedledum and Tweedledee. In: *Alice's Adventures in Wonderland and Through the Looking Glass.* London: Bloomsbury Publishing; 2010. Ch 4. p. 256.

21 Rowe M. Wait time: slowing down may be a way of speeding up. *Journal of Teacher Education.* 1986; **7**: 43–50.

22 Tennyson A. Break, break, break. In: Ricks C, editor. *Selected Poems.* London: Penguin Classics; 2007. p. 89.

23 Pendleton D, Scofield T, Tate P, *et al. The Consultation: an approach to learning and teaching.* Oxford: Oxford University Press; 1984. By permission of OUP.

24 Salmon P. The potentially somatizing effect of clinical consultation. *CNS Spectrums.* 2006; **11**(3): 190–200.

25 Bendix T. *The Anxious Patient.* London: Churchill Livingstone; 1982. pp. 9–17.

26 Ibid.

27 Chaucer G. *The Canterbury Tales. General Prologue.* Mann J, editor. London: Penguin Classics; 2005. p. 19.

28 Rutter M, Cox A. Psychiatric interviewing techniques: I. Methods and Measures. *Br J Psychiatry.* 1981; **138**: 273–82.

29 Silverman J, Kurtz S, Draper J. *Skills for Communicating with Patients.* 3rd ed. London: Radcliffe Publishing; 2013.

30 Agur A, Dalley A. *Grant's Atlas of Anatomy.* Philadelphia, PA: Lippincott Williams & Wilkins; 2012.

31 Coleridge ST. The rime of the ancyent marinere. In: Stafford F, editor. Wordsworth W, Coleridge ST. *Lyrical Ballads: 1798 and 1802.* Oxford: Oxford University Press; 2013. p. 5.

32 Holub M. *The Dimension of the Present Moment: essays.* London: Faber & Faber; 1990. p. 6.

33 Ibid.

34 Yeats WB. He wishes for the cloths of heaven. In: *The Collected Poems of W.B. Yeats.* Ware: Wordsworth Editions; 2008. p. 59.

35 Byrne PS, Long BE. *Doctors Talking to Patients.* London: HMSO; 1976.

36 Beckman HB, Frankel RM. The effect of physician behaviour on the collection of data. *Ann Intern Med.* **101**(5): 692–6.

37 Bendix T, op. cit.

38 Ibid.

39 Fox K. *Watching the English: the hidden rules of English behaviour.* London: Hodder & Stoughton; 2004.

40 Rowe M, op. cit.

41 Rutter M, Cox A, op. cit.

42 Ibid.

43 Bendix T, op. cit.

44 Austen J. Emma. In: *The Works of Jane Austen.* London: Hamlyn; 1976. p. 826.

45 Beauchamp TL, Childress JF. *Principles of Biomedical Ethics.* 3rd ed. Oxford: Oxford University Press; 1989.

46 Gillon R. Medical ethics: four principles plus attention to scope. *BMJ.* 1994; **309**(6948): 184–8.

47 De Waal E. *A Life-Giving Way: a commentary on the Rule of St Benedict.* London: Geoffrey Chapman; 1995.

48 Gazda GM, Balzer FJ, Childers WC, *et al. Human Relations Development: a manual for educators.* 7th ed. Boston, MA: Allyn and Bacon; 2005.

49 Ovid. Narcissus and Echo. In: *Metamorphoses: a new verse translation.* Book 3. Raeburn D, translator. London: Penguin Books; 2004.

50 Gibran K. *The Prophet.* London: William Heinemann; 1972. p. 73.

51 World Medical Association (WMA). *Declaration of Geneva.* (Amended 1968 and 1983.) London: WMA; 1949.

52 Helman CG. Disease versus illness in general practice. *J R Coll Gen Pract.* 1981; **31**(230): 548–52.

53 Barrie JM. *Peter Pan.* Chapter 1. Peter Breaks Through. London: Penguin Classics; 1995. pp. 6–7.

54 Ibid.

55 Department of Health and Social Security (DHSS). *Inequalities in Health: report of a research working group.* (The Black Report). London: DHSS; 1980.

56 Ibid.

57 Shaw GB. *The Doctor's Dilemma: a tragedy.* London: Penguin Classics; 1987.

58 National Institute for Health and Care Excellence. *NICE 'Do Not Do' Recommendations.* Available at: www.nice.org.uk/usingguidance/donotdorecommendations/index.jsp (accessed 14 December 2013).

59 Audit Commission. *Reducing Spending on Low Clinical Value Treatments. Health briefing.* London: Audit Commission Publishing Team; 2011. Available at: www.audit-commission.gov.uk/technicaldirectory/downloads/vfm/20101208localsavingsreview guide_reducingexpenditure.pdf (accessed 14 December 2013).

60 Shakespeare W. *Macbeth.* Act 5, scene 3. In: Wells S, Taylor G, editors. *William Shakespeare The Complete Works.* Oxford: Oxford University Press; 1988. p. 997.

61 Forster EM. *Howards End.* London: Penguin Modern Classics; 1971.

62 Grimm JL, Grimm W. *Kinder und Hausmärchen* [Household Tales]. Gütersloh: Bertelsmann; 1890.

63 Silverman J, Kurtz S, Draper J, op. cit.

64 Hall JA, Roter DL, Katz NR. Meta-analysis of correlates of provider behaviour in medical encounters. *Med Care.* 1988; **26**: 657-75.

65 Tuckett D, Boulton M, Olsen C, *et al. Meetings Between Experts: an approach to sharing ideas in medical consultations.* London: Tavistock; 1985.

66 Silverman J, Kurtz S, Draper J, op. cit.

67 Britten N, Stevenson FA, Barry CA, *et al.* Misunderstandings in prescribing decisions in general practice: qualitative study. *BMJ.* 2000; **320**(7233): 484–8.

68 Charles C, Gafni A, Whelan T. How to improve communication between doctors and patients: learning more about the decision making context is important. *BMJ.* 2000; **320**(7244): 1220–1.

69 Ibid.

70 Tolstoy L. *War and Peace* (1868), Vol. 1, Part 1, Chapter 25. London: Penguin Classics; 2007. p. 108.

71 Osler W. *Aequanimitas: with other addresses to medical students, nurses and practitioners of medicine.* 2nd ed. Chapter 3: Teacher and Student. Philadelphia, PA: P. Blakiston's Son & Co; 1910. p. 87.

72 Kurtz S, Silverman J, Draper J. *Teaching and Learning Communication Skills in Medicine.* 2nd ed. Oxford: Radcliffe Publishing; 2004.

73 Doll R, Hill AB. Smoking and carcinoma of the lung: preliminary report. *BMJ.* 1950; **2**(4682): 739–48.

74 Hobbes T. *Leviathan: revised student edition.* Tuck R, editor. Chapter 13: The Naturall Condition of Mankind. Cambridge: Cambridge University Press; 1996. p. 89.

75 Newton I. *Letter to Robert Hooke.* 1676.

76 Goll J. *Undergraduate Thesis.* Princeton, NJ: Princeton University.

77 Balint E, Norell JS, editors. *Six Minutes for the Patient: interactions in general practice consultation.* Chapter 1 Research in Psychotherapy. London: Tavistock Publications; 1973. p. 1.

78 Ibid.

79 Berne E. *Games People Play: the psychology of human relationships.* London: Penguin Books; 1970.

80 Da Vinci L. *The Notebooks of Leonardo da Vinci.* Richter I, editor. Oxford: Oxford University Press; 1952.

81 Working Party of the Royal College of General Practitioners, op. cit.

82 Spence J. The need for understanding the individual as part of the training and function of doctors and nurses. In: *The Purpose and Practice of Medicine.* London: Oxford University Press; 1960. pp. 273–4. By permission of OUP.

83 Working Party of the Royal College of General Practitioners, op. cit.

84 Medawar P. *The Art of the Soluble: creativity and originality in science.* London: Penguin Books; 1969.

85 Balint M, op. cit.

86 Balint E, Norell JS, editors. *Six Minutes for the Patient: interactions in general practice consultation.* London: Tavistock Publications; 1973.

87 Ibid.

88 Ibid.

89 Shakespeare W. Hamlet. Act 2, scene 2. In: Wells S, Taylor G, editors. *William Shakespeare The Complete Works.* Oxford: Oxford University Press; 1988. p. 666.

90 Hochbaum GM. Why people seek diagnostic X-rays. *Public Health Rep.* 1956; **71**(4): 377–80.

91 Becker MH. The health belief model and personal health behaviour. *Health Educ Monogr.* 1974; **2**: 324–473.

92 Becker MH, Maiman LA. Sociobehavioral determinants of compliance with medical care recommendations. *Med Care.* 1975; **13**(1): 10–24.

93 Heron J. Introduction to *Helping the Client: a creative practical guide.* London: Sage Publications; 2001. pp. 4–7.

94 Eliot T. *Four Quartets.* London: Faber and Faber; 1959. p. 39.

95 Byrne PS, Long BE, op. cit.

96 Stott NC, Davis RH. The exceptional potential in each primary care consultation. *J R Coll Gen Pract.* 1979; **29**(201): 201–5.

97 Ibid.

98 Helman CG. Disease versus illness in general practice. *J R Coll Gen Pract.* 1981; **31**(230): 548–52.

99 Ibid.

100 Cassell EJ. *The Healer's Art: a new approach to the doctor-patient relationship.* Harmondsworth: Penguin Books; 1978.

101 Helman CG. op. cit.

102 Helman C. Hieroglyphics. In: *Irregular Numbers of Beasts and Birds: the slow buzz of exhausted insects.* Florence, MA: Quale Press; 2006. p. 15.

103 Pendleton D, Scofield T, Tate P, *et al.* op. cit.

104 Neighbour R. *The Inner Consultation.* 2nd ed. Oxford: Radcliffe Publishing; 2004.

105 Cohen-Cole S. *The Medical Interview: the three function approach.* St Louis, MO: Mosby; 1991.

106 Silverman JD, Draper J, Kurtz SM. The inhumanity of medicine: interpersonal and communication skills can be taught. *BMJ.* 1995; **310**(6978): 527.

107 Kurtz S, Silverman J, Draper J, op. cit.

108 Silverman J, Kurtz S, Draper J, op. cit.

109 Brodie H. Foreword. In: Greenhalgh T, Hurwitz B, editors. *Narrative Based Medicine: dialogue and discourse in clinical practice.* London: BMJ Books; 1988. p. xiii.

110 Bayliss R. Chapter 8. Pain narratives. In: Greenhalgh T, Hurwitz B, editors. *Narrative Based Medicine: dialogue and discourse in clinical practice.* London: BMJ Books; 1988. p. 75.

111 Heath I. Chapter 9. Following the story: continuity of care in general practice. In: Greenhalgh T, Hurwitz B, editors. *Narrative Based Medicine: dialogue and discourse in clinical practice.* London: BMJ Books; 1988. p. 83.

112 Ibid. p. 86.

113 Launer J. Chapter 10. Narrative and mental health in primary care. In: Greenhalgh T, Hurwitz B, editors. *Narrative Based Medicine: 3 and discourse in clinical practice.* London: BMJ Books; 1988. p. 95.

114 Moulton L. *The Naked Consultation.* Oxford: Radcliffe Publishing; 2007.

115 Stuart M, Liebermann J. *The Fifteen Minute Hour: therapeutic talk in primary care.* Oxford: Radcliffe Publishing; 2008.

116 Naidoo P, Monkley C. *Consultations Skills for the New MRCGP: practice cases for the CSA and COT.* Banbury: Scion Publishing; 2009.

117 Ibid.

118 Ibid.

Index

Entries in **bold** refer to figures.

CPD with Radcliffe

You can now use a selection of our books to achieve CPD (Continuing Professional Development) points through directed reading.

We provide a free online form and downloadable certificate for your appraisal portfolio. Look for the CPD logo and register with us at: www.radcliffehealth.com/cpd